ERIKA,
HERE'S A BOOK TO HELP YOUR SEX LIFE.
HAPPY READING!
Jodi

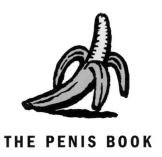

THE PENIS BOOK

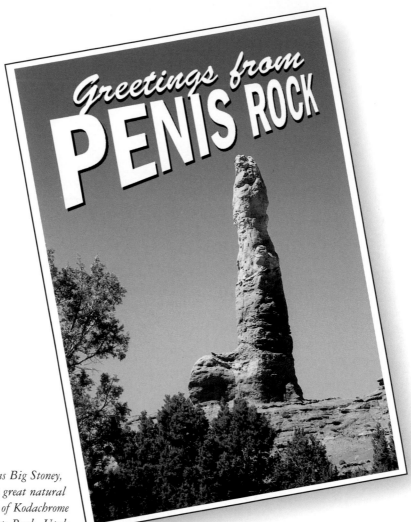

Greetings from **PENIS ROCK**

Also known as Big Stoney, it's one of the great natural wonders of Kodachrome Basin State Park, Utah.

THE PENIS BOOK

Joseph Cohen

KÖNEMANN

Produced by
Fresh Ideas Daily
New York City

Designed by
Tom Dolle Design
New York City

Publishing Director: Peter Feierabend
Production Director: Deltev Schaper
©1999 Joseph Cohen
©1999 Könemann Verlagsgesellschaft mbH

Könemann Verlagsgesellschaft mbH
Bonner Str. 126, D-50968
Cologne , Germany

Printed in Hong Kong
ISBN: 3-8290-2186-0

10 9 8 7 6 5 4 3 2 1

You have one.

You want one.

You love them.

You hate them...

The penis.

It's hard to imagine
that something tinier
than a chihuahua
can stir up so many
emotions,
escapades,
steamy page-turners,
phone sex businesses,
visits to the shrink,
babies,
dirty jokes,
sleepless nights,
dreamy sighs,
lies,
embarrassed giggles.

And so much fun.

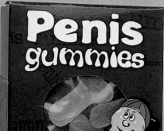

Penis gummies

Soft Chewy Gummies
in 2 Fruity Flavors

Net Wt. 5.3oz. (150g)

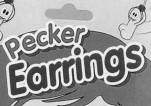

Pecker Earrings

(IT,S REALISTIC)   IMAGINARY   (IT,S

LEG STRAP
2 FOOT COCK

STRAP COCK TO YOUR LEG
STICK UP BOTTOM OF PANTS,
BE SHOCKING
BE THE LIFE OF THE PARTY

Made in Hong Kong

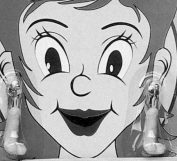

WIMPY WILLY
CANDLE

pd

Jelly
Chocolate Dream

Multi-Speed

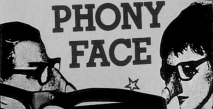

PHONY FACE

EVER MADE

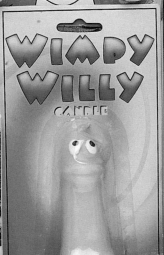

WIN
SC
Ne

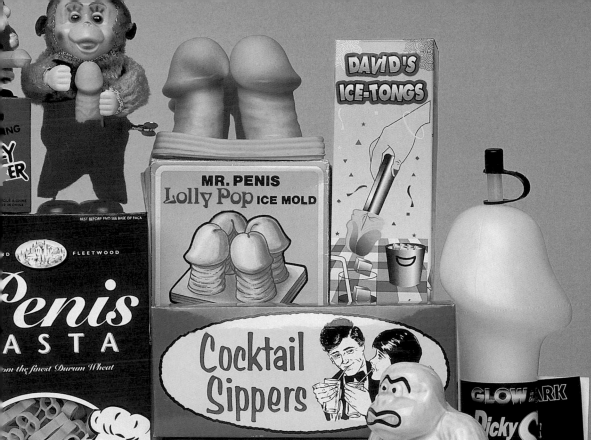
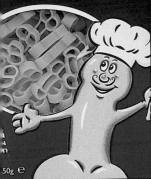
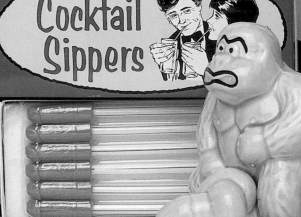
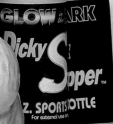

IT'S THE MOMENT OF TRUTH.

TIME TO SEE HOW YOU MEASURE UP WITH

THE REAL MEN OF THE WORLD.

Step right up

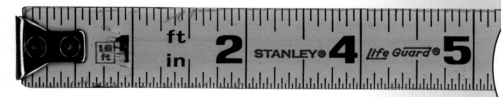

ft
in

2 STANLEY® 4 life Guard® 5

7

Most guys dream of sporting a long, thick porno porker instead of their trusty cocktail frank. Forget it. If you're like most men, no yardstick is necessary for this assignment. While there are some amazing exceptions to the ruler, here's the law of averages: **The average length of a flaccid penis is 3.7 inches, with a diameter of 1.25 inches. The average length of an erect penis is 5.1 inches, with a diameter of 1.6 inches. Penises usually reach their manly max by the time a male turns 17.**

WEET REVENGE. The shorter a guy's penis, the bigger it blossoms. Many chaps whose members are in the three-inch range when flaccid can look forward to organs that double in size when fully erect. Their hunkier buddies, on the other hand, almost never experience such generous growth...although they're still ahead of the game.

IG NOSE, BIG HOSE? Not necessarily. While we've all heard tales about beefy hands, noses and earlobes being surefire

6

drop your pants.

MADE IN U.S.A. **10** APP'D 339 TC **11** **14** **15**

signs that a huge dick is waiting in the wings, thousands of measurements over the years show no correlation. Penis size is very much a product of heredity and genetics, not the size of your loafers.

THE INCREDIBLE SHRINKING DICK.

Fear, stress and icy ocean water will all shrink a penis down to grade-school dimensions. During annual physical exams, approximately one-third of all males will feel a need to explain their diminished equipment, uttering something like: "Doc, it's really a lot bigger when I get out of here."

BLOW OFF THE DUST AND USE IT.

It's incredibly beneficial to keep your pecker sexually (and safely) active, most urologists agree. Erections fill your penis with oxygen-rich blood, and oxygen is essential for the survival of the smooth muscle tissue within the arteries of your ding-dong. A shortage of oxygen can eventually lead to a build-up of collagen, making erections a sweet memory. So use that tool!

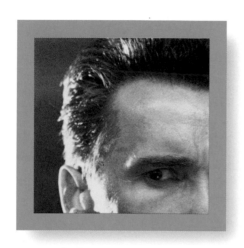

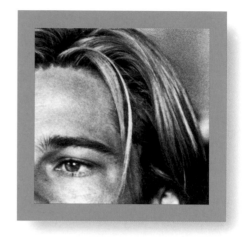

Schwarzenegger
has a long one...

Brad Pitt
has a short one...

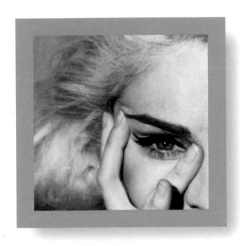

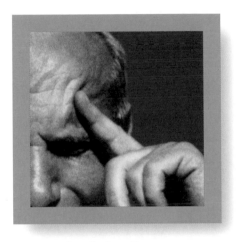

Madonna
doesn't have one...

And the Pope
never uses his.

WHAT IS IT?

ANSWER: A LAST NAME

9

Want a penis that's

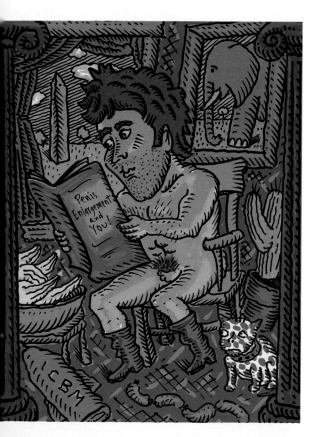

Call it equal opportunity. For decades, women have been adding glorious inches to their breasts. It was inevitable that guys would get their favorite toy tinkered with, too. Ads for penis enlargement services are everywhere, including a slew of sites on the Web complete with eye-opening before and after pictures.

Surgeons, smarting from the pittance that insurance companies are doling out for ornery arteries and gallbladders, are sniffing out a brave new world. And a gold mine from insecure peacocks. Their brochures are impressive, filled with glowing testimonials from born-again hunks. And look at those penises. Hefty, hanging tributes to the brilliance of "My son, the doctor."

Assuming your ticker and other vital signs check out okay—and you've brought along a certified check for a few

10

two inches longer?

grand (credit cards are always welcomed)— you and shorty are headed for the big time. While you're under a general anesthetic, your doctor will make a small incision just above the base of the penis. Next, he'll cut the main suspensory ligaments that anchor the penis to your pubic bone, allowing the inch or so of penis that is normally inside your body to hang outside. (In case you're interested, this procedure was invented in China by a surgeon named Long.)

You're half-way there. Guys inevitably want a chunkier, girthier look, too. Most surgeons take care of this request by injecting purified fat, removed from the abdomen or lower thigh, under the skin around the shaft of the penis. Another enlarging technique is known as dermal graft augmentation. With this method, strips of skin with the fat on the undersurface are removed from the buttocks and placed under the skin of your penis.

The flip side of all this: there are lots of unhappy campers out there. In numerous cases, lengthening procedures are anything but that. Scar tissue forms where the ligament was cut, frequently causing the penis to retract, creating a shorter penis than when you started. Often, erections point straight out instead of up. Fat injections have also stirred up sad tales. After a few months, a man's body absorbs much of the fat, while remaining fat causes the penis to become bumpy and irregular in shape. Grafting may leave you with a bratwurst fantasy, but it can also leave you with serious scarring, loss of sensitivity, erection discomforts and, in some cases, impotence. It's no surprise a whole new breed of lawyers is specializing in penile malpractice.

A QUICK FIX WITHOUT SURGERY:

- Trim your pubic hair.
- Lose weight.
- Be happy with what you've got.

THE AVERAGE MALE...

between the ages of 15 and 60
will ejaculate 30 to 50 quarts of semen,
containing 350 to 500 billion sperm cells.

Average volume of ejaculate:	*0.5 to 1 teaspoon*
Chief ingredient:	*fructose*
Caloric content:	*5 calories per teaspoon*
Protein content:	*6 milligrams per teaspoon*
Average number of ejaculatory spurts:	*3 to 10*
Average speed of ejaculation:	*25 miles per hour*
Average interval of ejaculatory contractions:	*0.8 seconds*
Average duration of orgasm:	*4 seconds*
Farthest medically recorded ejaculation:	*11.7 inches*
Average number of sperm cells in ejaculate of a healthy man:	*200 to 600 million*
Average number in ejaculate of an infertile man:	*50 million*
Average swimming speed:	*1 to 4 millimeters per minute*

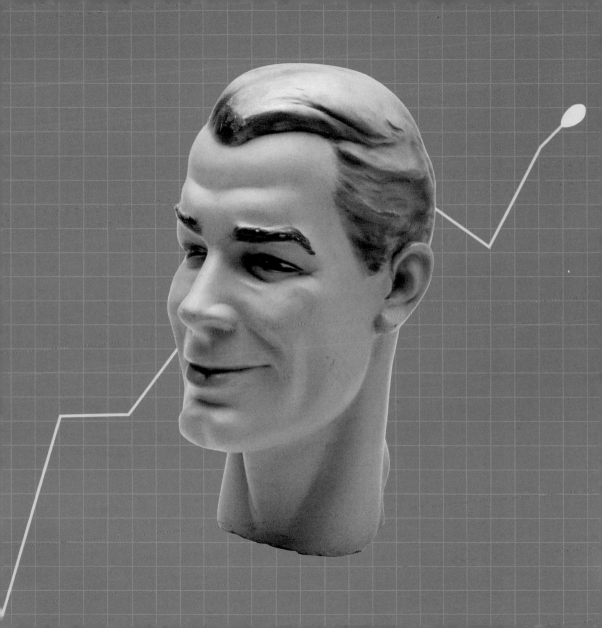

Actually, testicles are about 4°F cooler than the rest of a man's body temperature, providing the ideal climate for copious sperm production. (Avoid hot tubs and tight bikini underwear if you're trying to conceive.) ✳ About 90 percent of the male hormone testosterone originates in the testicles before it enters the bloodstream and travels throughout the body. ✳ European testicles tend to weigh about twice as much as their Chinese cousins. ✳ To prevent a life-long collision course, the left testicle hangs lower in about 85% of the male population and is usually a bit larger. ✳ When taking an oath, our biblical ancestors would place their hands over the testicles of a witness to indicate their sincerity and honesty. Words like "testify" and "testament" all derive from this unique association. ✳ Recent studies from England indicate that guys with large testicles had sex about 30% more often than their smaller-balled brothers and were more likely to cheat on their partners. ✳ Eunuchs of the Chinese Imperial Court often carried their pickled testicles in jars which they displayed around their necks. ✳ Testicular cancer has the highest cure rate of any cancer when it is detected in its early stage. Monthly self-exams are encouraged and should take place after a shower when the scrotal skin is relaxed. ✳ While testicles deserve tender loving care, men also love having their balls squeezed, sucked, slapped and tugged. He'll let you know when you're going too far. ✳ Each September, Montana's Original Testicle Festival serves more than 4,500 pounds of deep-fried bull's testicles, better known as Mountain Oysters. No bones. Dig right in. ✳ Vary your vocabulary for a rich conversation: Family Jewels, Nuts, Clangers, Spunk Holders, Jizz Sack, Cojones, Plums, Kiwis, Hairy Prunes, Fuzz Balls, Mike & Mo and the Melon Boys are all lively substitutes.

Great Balls Of

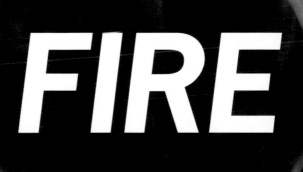

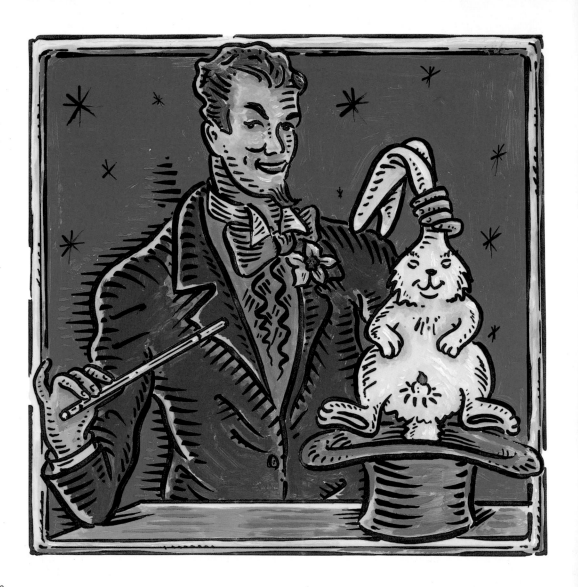

ABRACADABRA
Potency in a Pill

Who would have guessed that a pill originally developed to treat heart disease would spread boner mania across the globe?

For the world's 140 million men who suffer from long-term erectile dysfunction, Viagra is the closest thing yet to a fountain of youth. It works by relaxing smooth muscle cells in the penis, making it easier for the penis to engorge with blood and maintain an erection.

Just set your clock/cock to about one hour before desired lift-off. Swallow your pill. And gather up your sexiest CDs. You might want a few, since Viagra enables many men to experience erections for up to four hours. That's good news for premature ejaculators, grateful for a second chance. And for their female partners, who are finally getting the satisfying, long-distance ride they deserve (a lot longer than the average tryst of $1^1/_2$ minutes).

THINK BIG. By the year 2000, Viagra will be available on a worldwide. Already, it's the most successful new drug in the history of medicine.

THINK PINK. Viagra for women? Promising research from Europe suggests that Viagra can help restore a woman's sexual responsiveness by allowing more blood to flow into the vagina, particularly the clitoris—which is closer to a penis than most guys would like to admit.

WRITER'S CRAMP. Many doctors have their Viagra prescriptions embossed on a rubber stamp, smart idea for a pill that was prescribed 340,000 times in one week alone.

COMING. Plenty of competition...a potency pill that takes effect within 15 minutes, a rub-on gel for a dependable pick-me-up and a potency restorer nasal spray.

DAN QUAYLE ON VIAGRA: "I've been using this stuff for one week and nothing! It's the worst suppository I've ever tried."

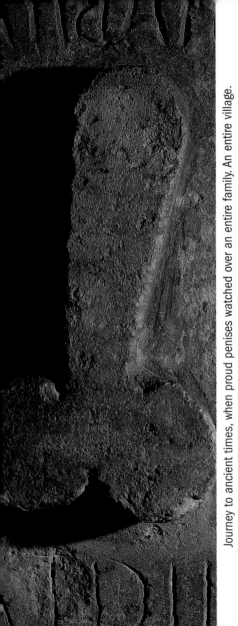

Journey to ancient times, when proud penises watched over an entire family. An entire village.

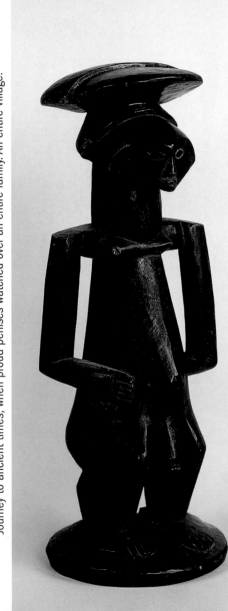

Here were the symbols of birth, of harvests greater than the year before, of power over enemies and the unknown.

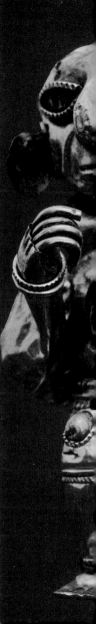

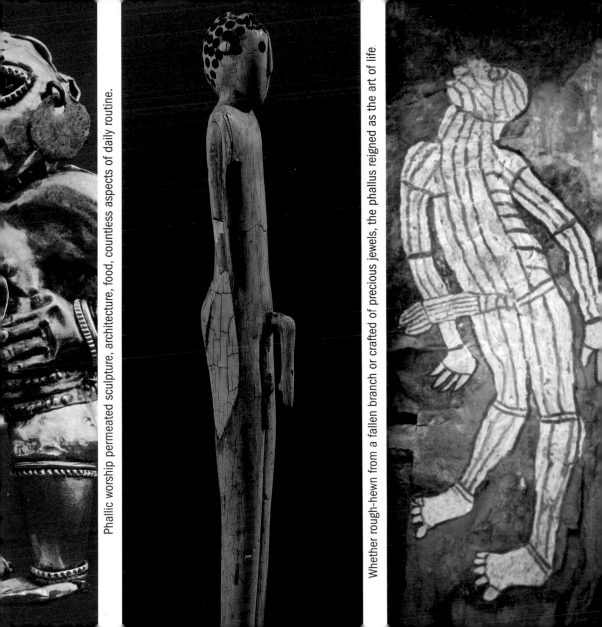

Phallic worship permeated sculpture, architecture, food, countless aspects of daily routine.

Whether rough-hewn from a fallen branch or crafted of precious jewels, the phallus reigned as the art of life

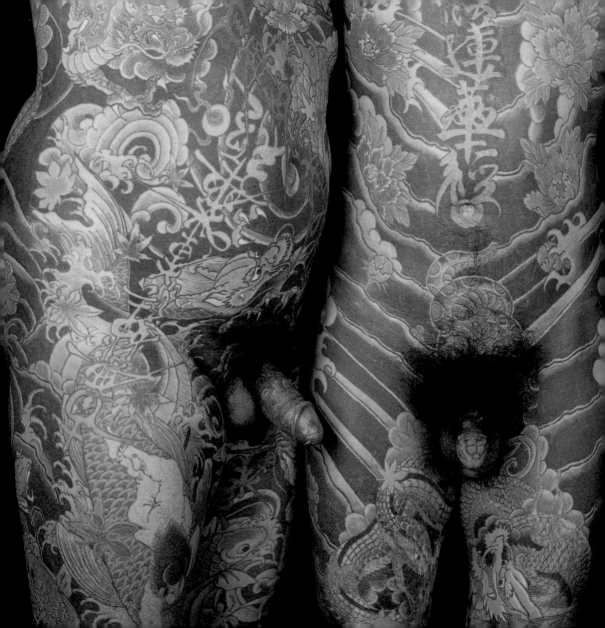

Taboo

They're called *Irezumi*, a rather secretive group of Japanese men and women, often drawn from the underworld, who transform their bodies into living works of art. The penis is the last part of the anatomy to be tattooed and it's always the most painful procedure, with the tattoo master focusing on a tiny section per session.

Even after death, these adorned bodies continue to amaze. Some 300 half-body and full-body skins have been preserved in airtight frames and sold to museums and private collectors. Interested? A few years ago, a half-body tattoo was auctioned for $50,000.

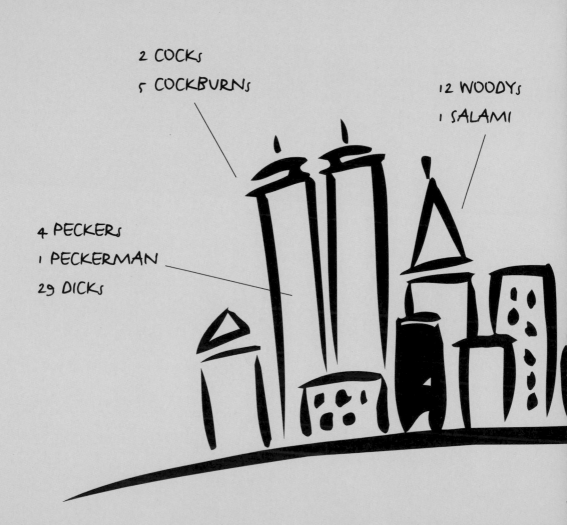

2 COCKs
5 COCKBURNs

12 WOODYs
1 SALAMI

4 PECKERS
1 PECKERMAN
29 DICKs

1 PRICKETT
4 HOSES
1 PISMAN
295 FRANKS

85 BALLS
1 BALLMAN
118 DONGS

124 WIENERS
4 HARDONS

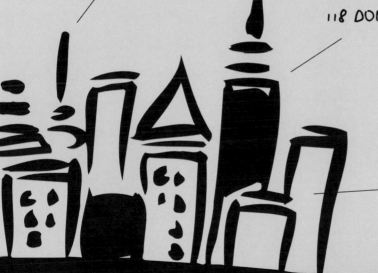

SCHWANZ ◀ GERMAN ANDER ◀ ARMENIAN

◀ BULGARIAN ▶ PISCHKA

PAJARITO

▲ CATALAN ZAKILA STAKU

▲ BASQUE NORWEGIAN ▶

◀ HEBREW

ZAYIN CHUJ

▲ CZECH

DUTCH ▶ KLOOTOOG AYIR

CAZZO CACETE ARABIC ▶

▲ ITALIAN ▲ PORTUGUESE ORTABACAK

TITTLINGUR KONTOL ◀ INDONESIAN ▲ TURKISH

▲ ICELANDIC

SWEDISH ▶ SNOPP

PULA

◀ ROMANIAN

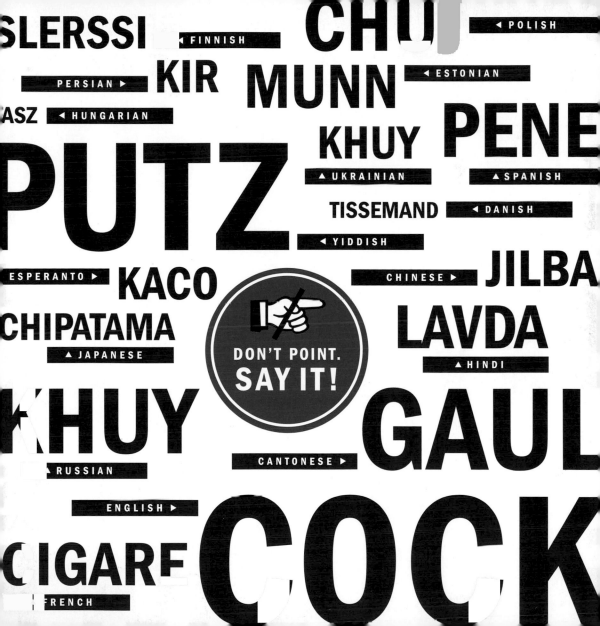

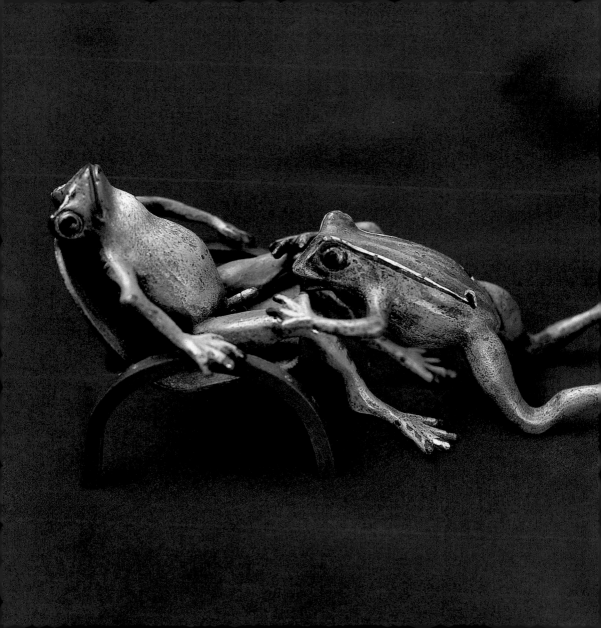

"Hey, hop on over to my pad
and I'll give you a blow job."

Somehow, it sounded more poetic when the ancient Greeks called it "playing the flute." Or when the Kama Sutra's scribes referred to it as *ambarchusi*, "sucking a mango."

Fellatio, from the Latin verb *fellare*, "to suck," has been around forever because it's such a simple and satisfying concept: a mouth on a penis. It can take place in an elevator, for the thrill of a quickie. Or on a satin-covered bed, with both partners pleasuring each other in a slurpy *soixante-neuf* co-mingle. Some men go absolutely wild being oral sexed while sitting buck naked on the kitchen counter. Many love it with their testicles pulled or a finger probing their anal opening. And then there are the Antarctic devotees, who crave the frosty zing of a mouth filled with ice cubes.

Many recipients find it impossible to achieve orgasm during oral sex, no matter how experienced the tongue flicker. No problem. Sucking is just one item on a grand sexual menu. And swallowing a hot load isn't everybody's idea of a fruit smoothie. Or a terrific example of safe sex.

PAINT YOUR
WALLS

Ivory Tower

Cockeyed
Curry

Manly
Mahogany

Mocha
Cream

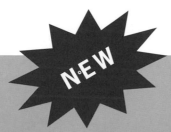

N·E·W

DELUXE FAUX FINISHES
Trickier...but worth it!

TO MATCH YOUR
PENIS

Prickly Pink

Raging Red

Honey Pie

Pouting
Purple

Pubissimo

Frecklehead

You're So Vein

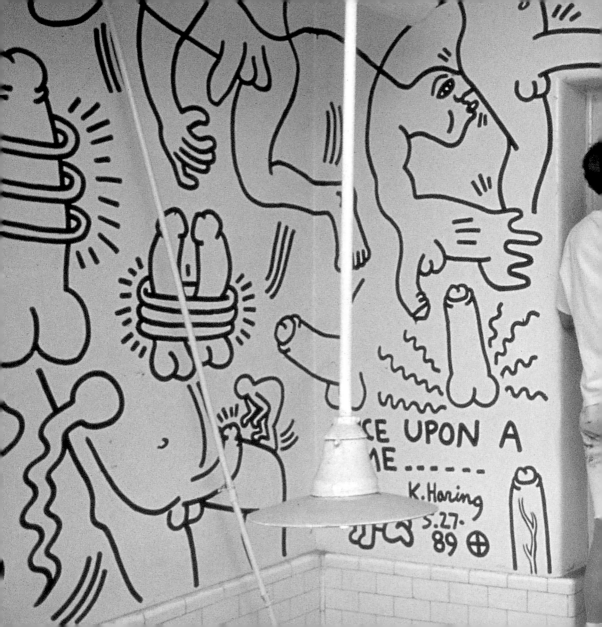

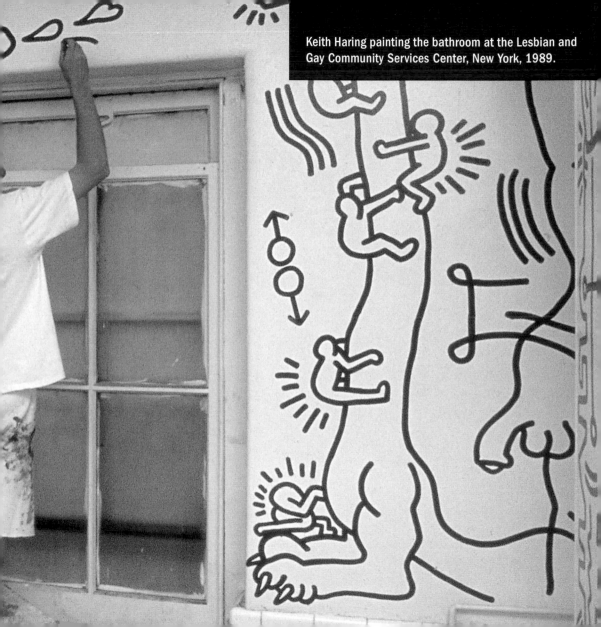

Keith Haring painting the bathroom at the Lesbian and Gay Community Services Center, New York, 1989.

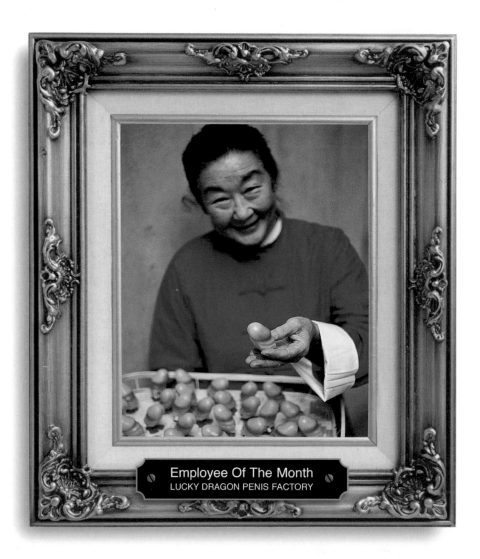

Employee Of The Month
LUCKY DRAGON PENIS FACTORY

"All day long make penis hop...make penis hop. Sometime foot fall off...spring pop and hit me in eye. More quick...make more happy penis boss say. Three hundred I make today...not enough...make more. May Wong at table next say her penis hop the biggest. You look like penis I say. She angry...later she laugh and laugh. I do job...go home and make egg drop soup for husband. No see his penis for three years."

—CHING LEE

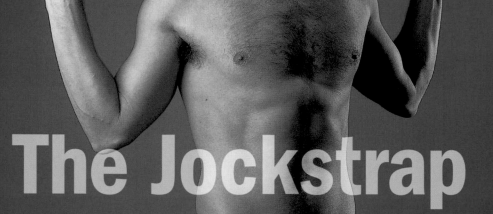

The Jockstrap

The average male will own six jockstraps from ages 12 to 60.

Jockstraps have been around since 1874. The Bike Web Manufacturing Company engineered an athletic supporter to provide relief for bicycle jockeys tortured by the cobblestone streets of Boston. The "bike jockey strap" soon became known as the "jock strap." And the business of genital protection was off and running.

Remember the embarrassment of asking dad to buy your first jockstrap for gym class. "Gotta protect those testicles, son" came a fatherly reply as he handed over a contraption that would add its tantalizing bouquet to your locker for the rest of the year.

Like, wow! For total protection, consider a bulletproof jockstrap. They're now available from various body armor companies for about $300. (Yes, bulletproof bras are also for sale.)

Into used jockstraps? You're not alone. The Web (search: athletic supporters) is filled with eclectic recyclers who like 'em with a sweaty pedigree.

Good news, gals. Savvy manufacturers are now featuring female protective cups designed to prevent injuries to *your* pelvic region. Current color: white. Victoria's Secret, take note.

"And now he's tiny, and soft like a little bud of life!"

D.H.Lawrence, *Lady Chatterly's Lover*

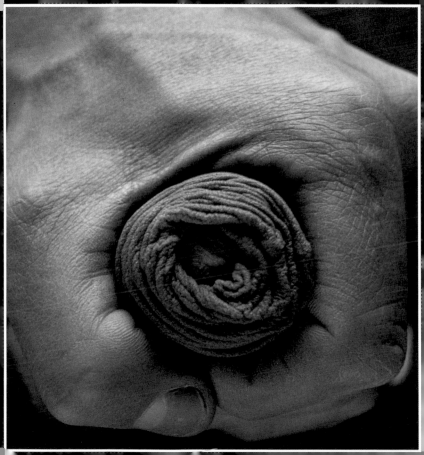

THE GREAT CIRCUMCISION
DEBATE

TWENTY-FIVE YEARS AGO, ALMOST 90 PERCENT OF AMERICA'S NEWBORN BOYS SAID FAREWELL TO FORESKINS THEY BARELY KNEW. TODAY, THAT SNIP, SNIP INTO MANHOOD IS ANYTHING BUT STANDARD PROCEDURE. FORESKINS ARE BACK IN A BIG WAY. ARGUMENTS PRO AND CON ARE PASSIONATE. TURTLENECK OR NOT, YOU DECIDE.

Let's hear it for tradition. If it was good enough for King David, Kirk Douglas and Prince Charles (who was attended to by London's premier *mohel*), why rock the boat? Advocates of circumcision cite a well-documented list of health benefits. For starters, circumcised infants are much less susceptible to urinary tract infection. The procedure virtually precludes penile cancer and eliminates balanoposthitis (an inflammation of the foreskin and glans usually caused by poor hygiene). Studies also reveal that circumcised men are at least twice as unlikely to catch herpes, syphilis and HIV during unsafe sex. And millions of folks just love that exposed "mushroom" head.

Anti-circumcision advocates are hardly sitting silently in the corner. They consider the procedure an inhumane act of genital mutilation (frequently performed without anesthesia), encoding the developing brain with pain instead of pleasure. Improved hygiene standards, they argue, have made foreskin-related diseases and infections increasingly rare. Advocates for intact penises assert that the numerous nerve endings in the foreskin and its gliding action contribute greatly to a man's sexual pleasure. It protects and lubricates the glans, which, with circumcision, often becomes less sensitive over the years. Their bottom line: Why would anyone want to discard the best part?

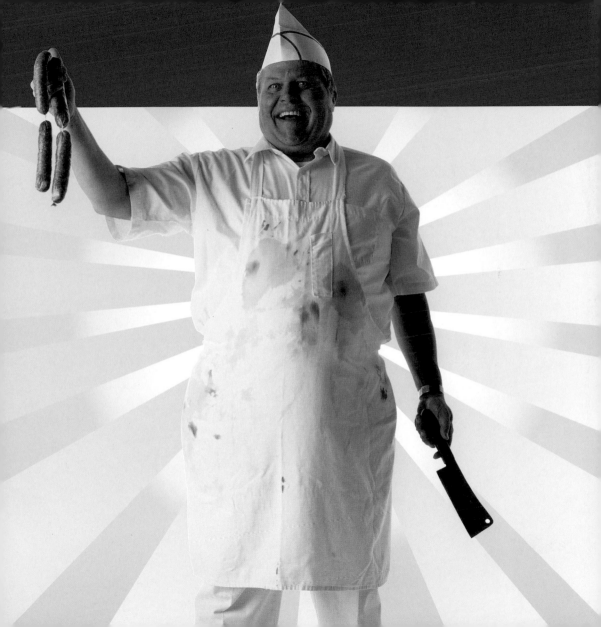

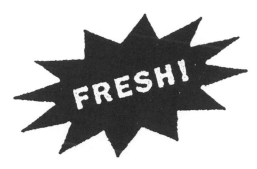

Foreskins for **Sale**

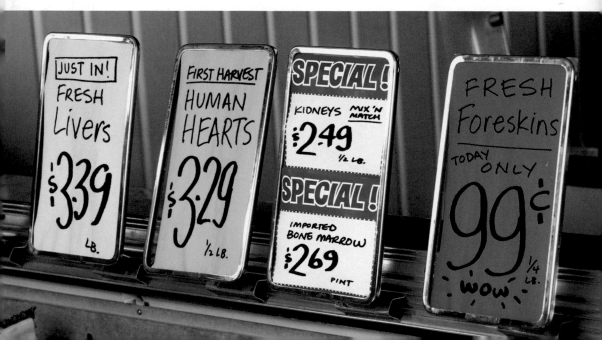

Ever wonder what hospitals do with a baby's foreskin once it's been removed? More often than not, this precious calamari isn't headed for the trash can.

Over the past two decades, hundreds of thousands of discarded foreskins have been sold to pharmaceutical companies and bio-research laboratories, which require young skin cells for clinical investigation and for the burgeoning field of artificial skin technology. One stamp-sized piece of foreskin contains enough genetic material to grow 200,000 units of faux skin.

For many, the promise of laboratory-created skin with living human epidermal and dermal cells is extraordinary, opening up major new avenues for the treatment of burns and wounds. For those who view circumcision as barbaric, the business of "harvesting" foreskins is an even greater insult. They ask: Who is the legal owner of a baby's foreskin after it has been cut off? And is it ethical for a hospital to sell a baby's foreskin without telling his parents—and keep the money?

...neeth, *v.t.* to smooth. [...]

smeg′mȧ, *n.* [Gr. *smēgma*, soap.] in physiology, a thick, cheesy secretion found under the prepuce in males and around the clitoris and labia minora in females.

smeg·mat′iç, *a.* being of the nature of [...]
[...] smelled *or* sm[...]

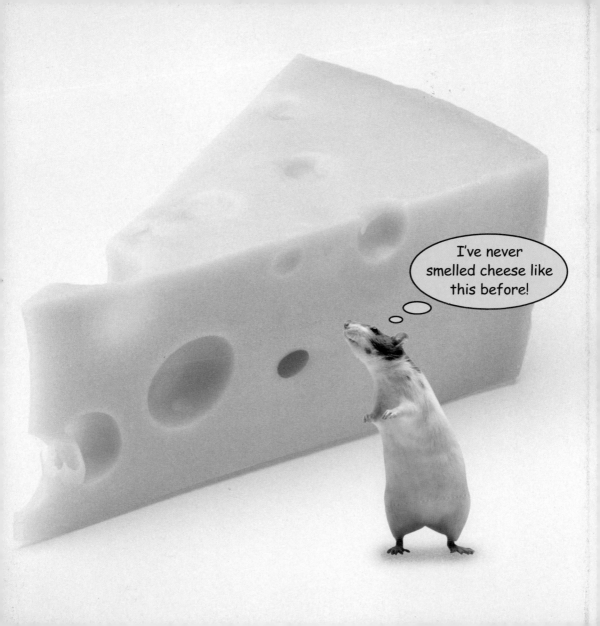

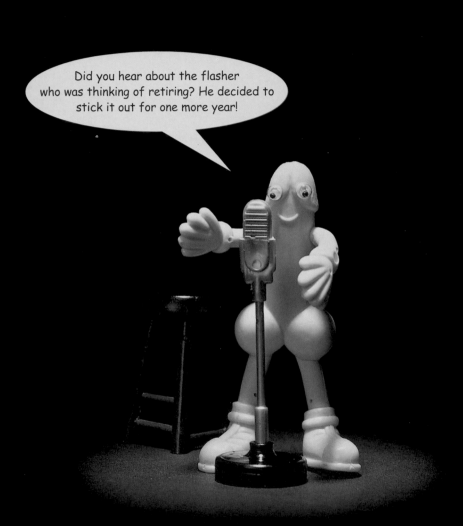

"God gave us a penis and a brain,
but only enough blood to run one at a time."

ROBIN WILLIAMS

THERE'LL BE NO

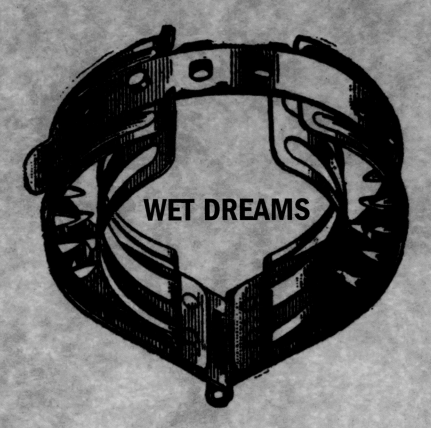

WET DREAMS

IN THIS HOUSE!

S omewhere around the age of 13, a boy's sperm factory kicks into high gear. Pumped with testosterone, young lads around the world find their nightly slumbers interrupted by the uncontrollable fireworks of *nocturnal emissions*, better known as wet dreams. Ah, the thrill of ejaculating (it's not uncommon for adolescents to have as many as 10 wet dreams a week). Oh, the confusion of explaining those cardboard-stiff sheets and pajama bottoms to mom.

In these so-called enlightened times, wet dreams and frequent masturbation urges are considered as natural a rite of passage as pimples and pubic hair. In the late nineteenth century, however, medical authorities in the United Sates and Europe decreed that the frequent spilling of semen would cause brains to grow dull and genitals to fall off. "The expenditure of the most vital fluids of the system" would surely bring early death.

These dire warnings gave birth to a brand new industry: the creation of anti-wet dream devices. In the user-friendliest contraptions, an expanding penis would cause an alarm to go off, averting seminal spillage. Pity the lad who went to bed wearing **The Timely Warning**, featured at left, patented in 1905 by Dr. Foote's Sanitary Bureau of New York. When an erection stirred, the menacing aluminum teeth were guaranteed to turn the sweetest dream into a living nightmare.

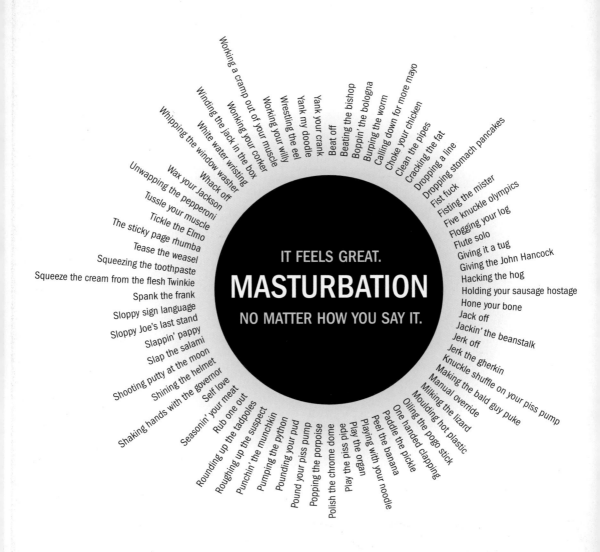

IT FEELS GREAT.

MASTURBATION

NO MATTER HOW YOU SAY IT.

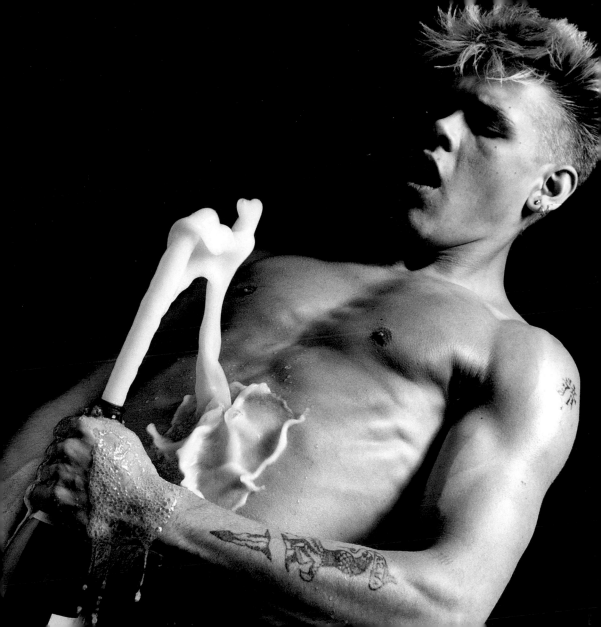

Latin For Lovers

The **urethra** is Route 66 of the penis world, stretching from the **bladder** to the penile opening. Urine and semen travel on it, but not at the same time.

The **prostate** is a male's G-spot, providing a surprising amount of pleasure when massaged. This chestnut-sized sex gland produces the thin, watery fluid that's a prime ingredient in semen. An enlarged prostate can be a real troublemaker, reducing a man's urine stream to a trickle. To stay clear of this and prostate cancer, a yearly digital rectal exam and PSA blood test are best bets.

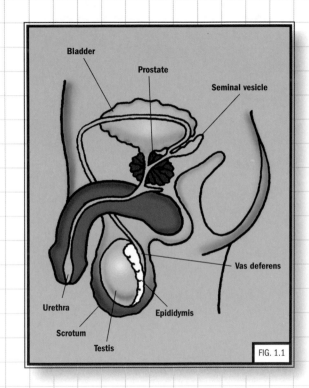

FIG. 1.1

The two **vas deferens** tubes conveying sperm from each testicle to the urethra are also the "vas" in vasectomy. In this common sterilizing procedure, a tiny segment of the tube is severed—end of the road for millions and millions of sperm.

The **epididymis** is a tube-filled mass at the back of the **testicles** where mature sperm enjoy a little siesta before embarking on their expedition up the vas deferens.

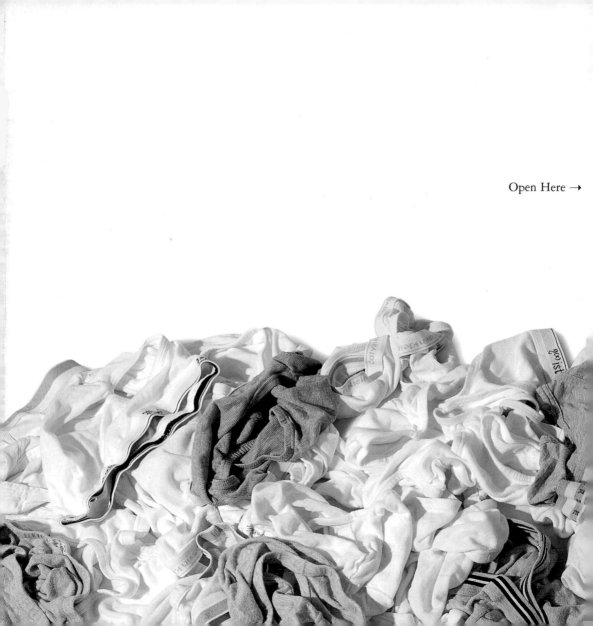

Open Here →

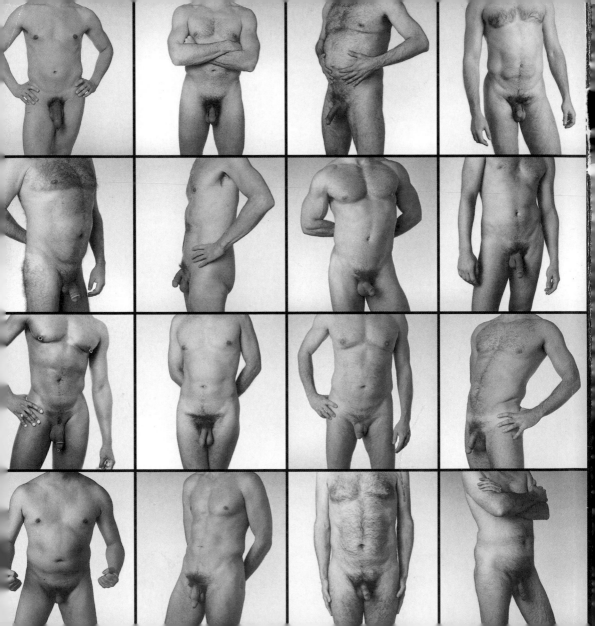

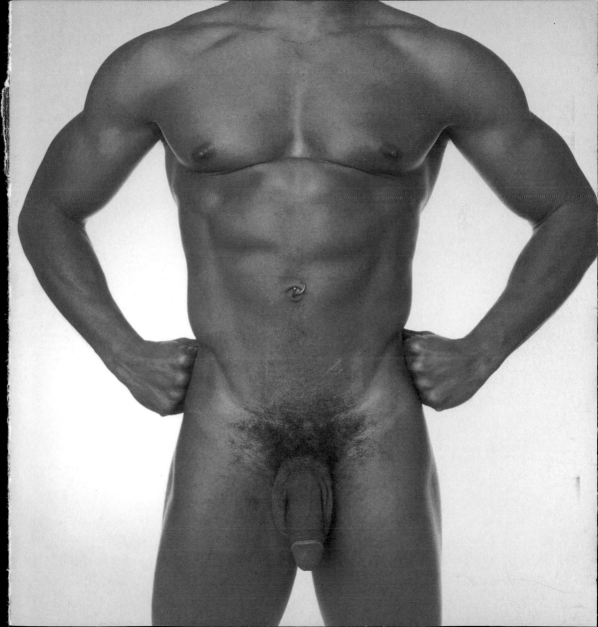

Thank you, **corpora cavernosa**. During sexual arousal, these two large spongy cylinders expand considerably as they fill with blood—about 10 times the amount of blood found in a flaccid penis. This hydraulic spectacle continues during sleep, also. Snoozing males usually experience hard-ons every 70 to 100 minutes, and sexy dreams have nothing to do with it. The penis is simply being reinvigorated with fresh oxygen and blood.

p.s.: there are no bones in the proverbial boner.

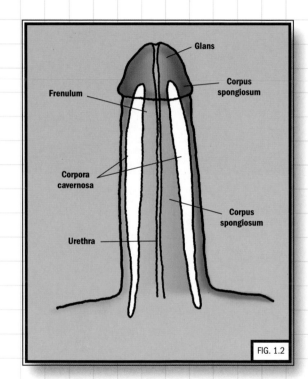

FIG. 1.2

Behold the **glans**, the head of the penis, consisting of soft tissue called **corpus spongiosum**. Glans is Latin for acorn.

Lots more **corpus spongiosum.**

It feels so good. The **frenulum** is a hotbed of sensitivity just below the glans on the underside of the penis.

DO IT YOURSELF

The dream goes something like this: You're naked at home, sitting on a chair with a rather sizable erection keeping you company. You bend your head down...and to your amazement, you effortlessly put your mouth over the head of your penis. "Boy, that was pretty easy", you say to yourself. "No big deal. I should do this more often!" And that's why they're called dreams. Unless you were born into a family of double-jointed circus performers from Minsk, sucking your own noodle is a tough assignment. But try to find a guy who hasn't tried it.

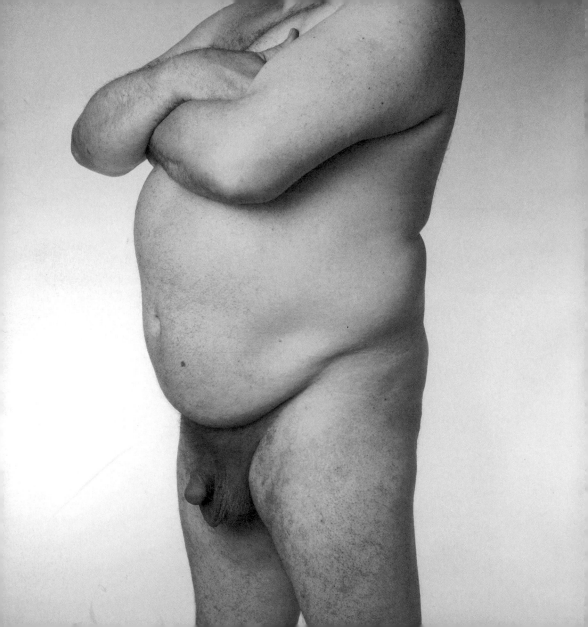

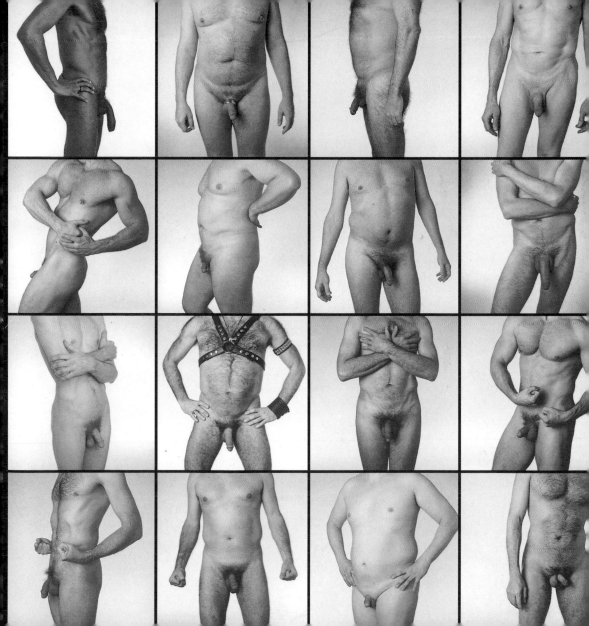

← Open Here

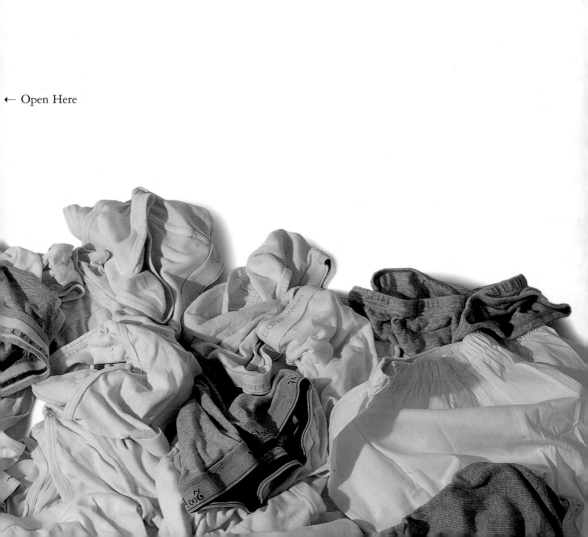

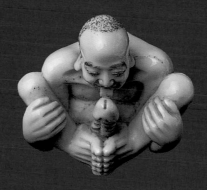

Once, when I was 17, I touched my dick with the tip of my nose. I'm 43 now
and sometimes I get a back spasm wiping my ass.

ALEX, LOUISVILLE

I would love to be able to suck myself off.
It's as queer as you can get without being queer.

ANTHONY, DALLAS

My girlfriend said she would take me to Acapulco if I could blow myself.
I got as far as Coney Island.

JULIO, NEW YORK

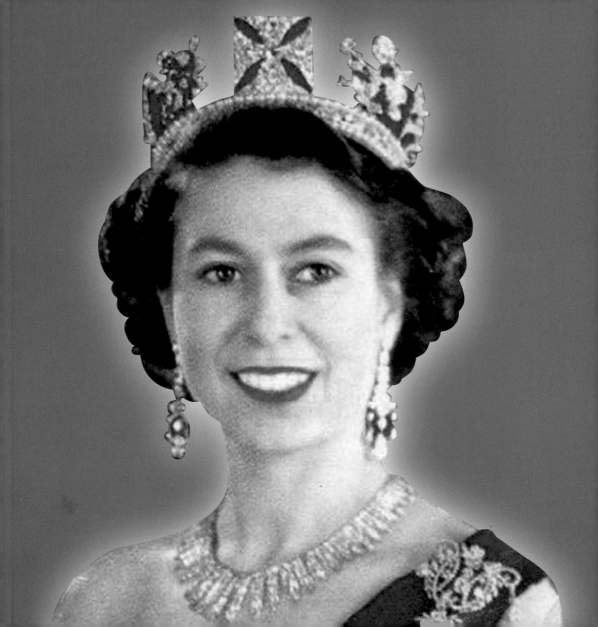

The Queen of England was visiting one of California's top hospitals and during her tour of the floors, she passed a room where a male patient was masturbating.

"Oh, my God," said the Queen, "that's disgraceful. What is the meaning of this?"

The doctor leading the tour explained: "I'm sorry your lady-ship, this man has a very serious condition where the testicles rapidly fill with semen. If he doesn't ejaculate five times a day, they'll explode and he would die instantly.

"How terrible," said the Queen.

On the next floor, they passed a room where a young nurse was giving a patient oral sex.

"Goodness," said the Queen, "what's happening in there?"

The Doctor replied: "Same problem, better health plan."

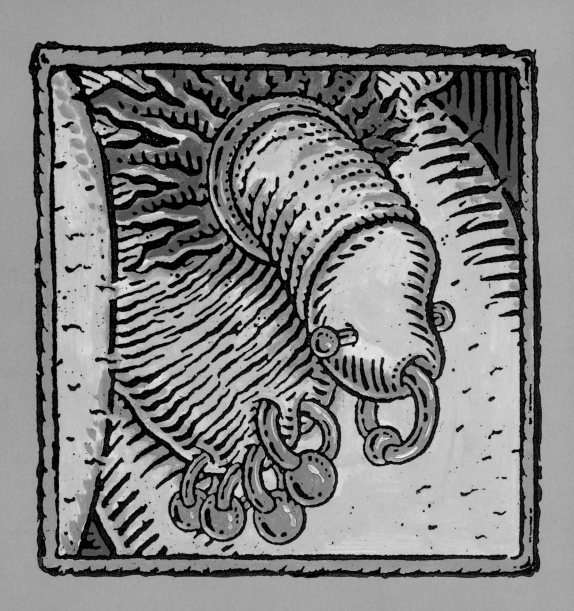

Prince Albert, you kinky devil.

"OUCH!"

It's a natural reaction if you've never seen a pierced penis before. And why would anyone name them after the husband of Queen Victoria?

Documents and diaries reveal that the penile heads of many upper-crust gentlemen during the Victorian era were pierced with a "dressing ring" used to firmly secure the male genitalia in either the left or right pant leg to prevent unsightly bulges. (Aren't you glad you were born a few years later?)

Today, bulges are celebrated and genital piercing is bigger than ever. Converts claim that piercing intensifies every orgasm for the male by stimulating the nerves that end in the glans of the penis. Their female partners rave about their intensified pleasure and heightened orgasms. In fact, there are many women who wouldn't dream of wasting their time with an unpierced wiener.

If you're considering costume jewelry south of the border, better know the lingo. The classic ring piercing the urethra and glans is called a *Prince Albert*. That barbell device through the head is called an *ampallang*, while a variation of this is called an *apadravya*. Add a bunch of flashy *hafadas* on your scrotum, *guiche* rings at the perineum and your favorite *cock rings* to lift and separate...and you're ready for anything. Including some amazing explanations every time you pass through airport security.

How much? Rates at the Gauntlet in New York City average $20 per genital piercing, with surgical stainless steel accessories starting at $25. A Prince Albert at Perforations in Brighton, England will set you back £20, including jewelry.

Hurt? While most guys reading this page are holding their crotches by now, Prince Alberts really aren't that painful...less of a zap than getting one's nipples pierced.

Peeing suggestions? Careful. Your straight stream of the past will now look like a watering can. Get close to the bowl. And those first few whizzes are sure to be stingers.

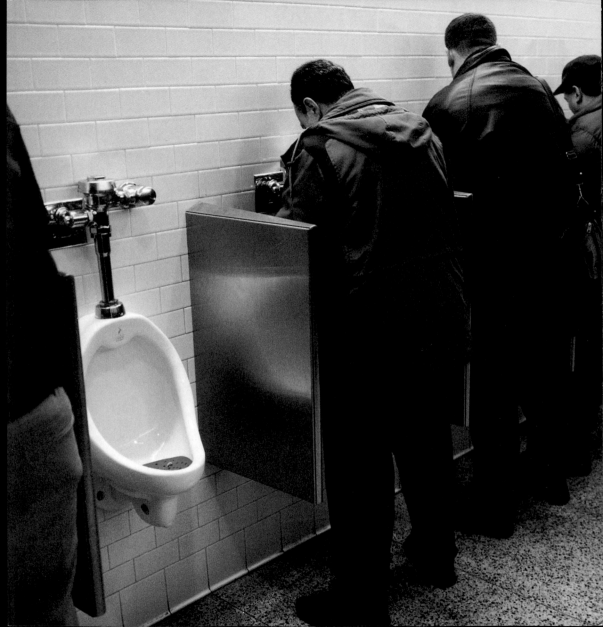

Urinal Etiquette

Refrain from whistling "The Man I Love" while peeing.

Avoid the temptation of saying: "Nice watch you got there."

If you must fart, don't make it a long-winded affair.

On those rare occasions when you have to use the little boy's urinal,
do not get on your knees.

Should you sense the guy next to you is piss shy, never comment:
"It's all in your head."

Be courteous when people are standing behind you.
Shake no more than three times.

Don't hog the hot air dryer trying to dry those last drops
on your pants. Hide your little puddle with a highly regarded
newspaper or a fine cashmere topcoat.

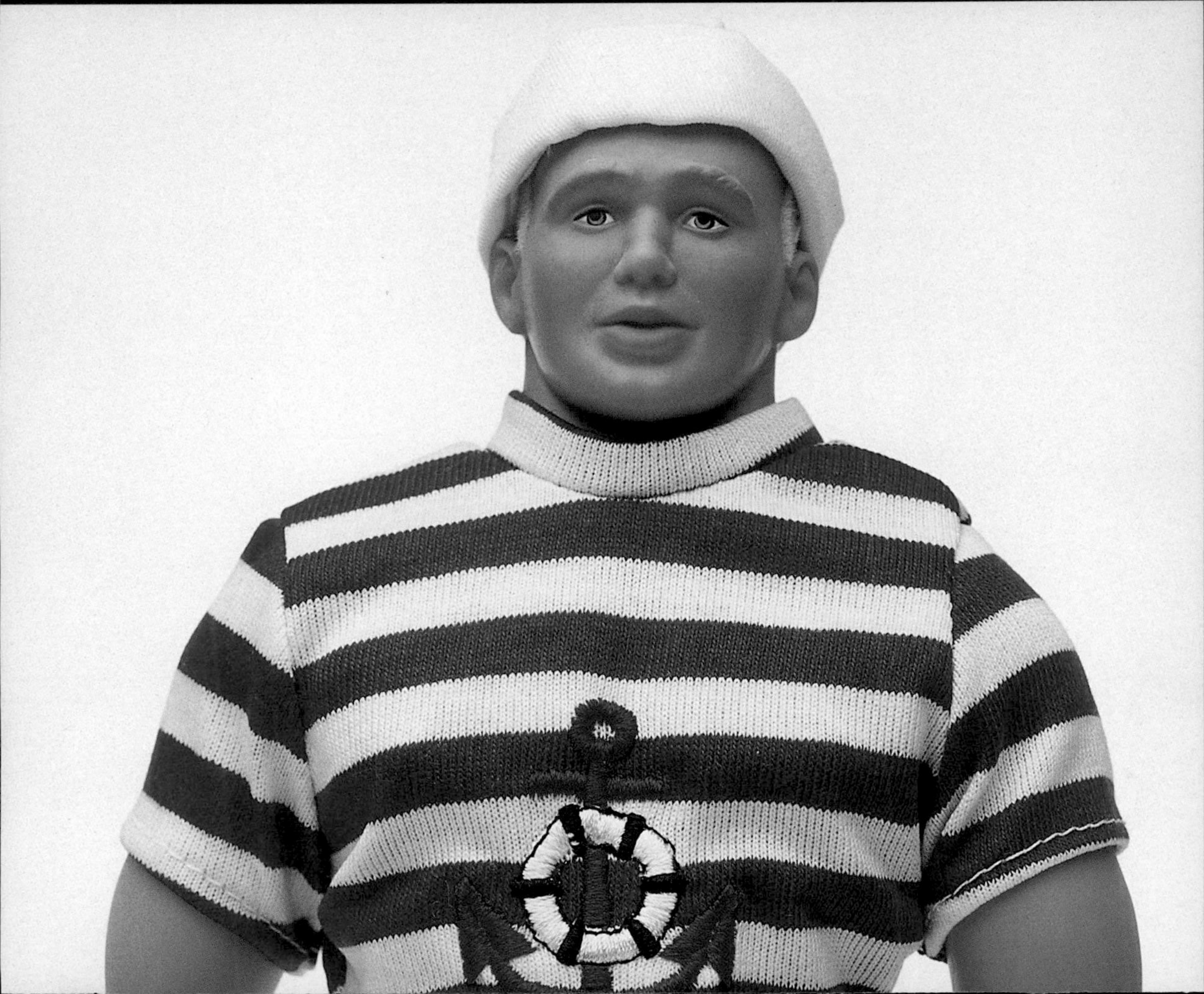

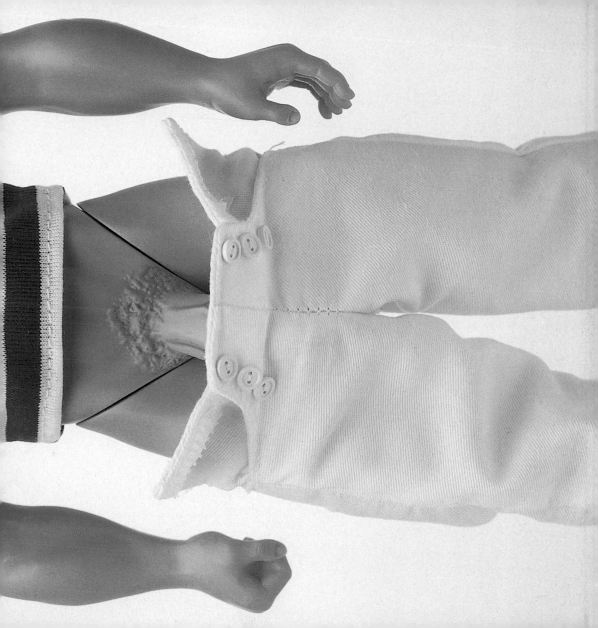

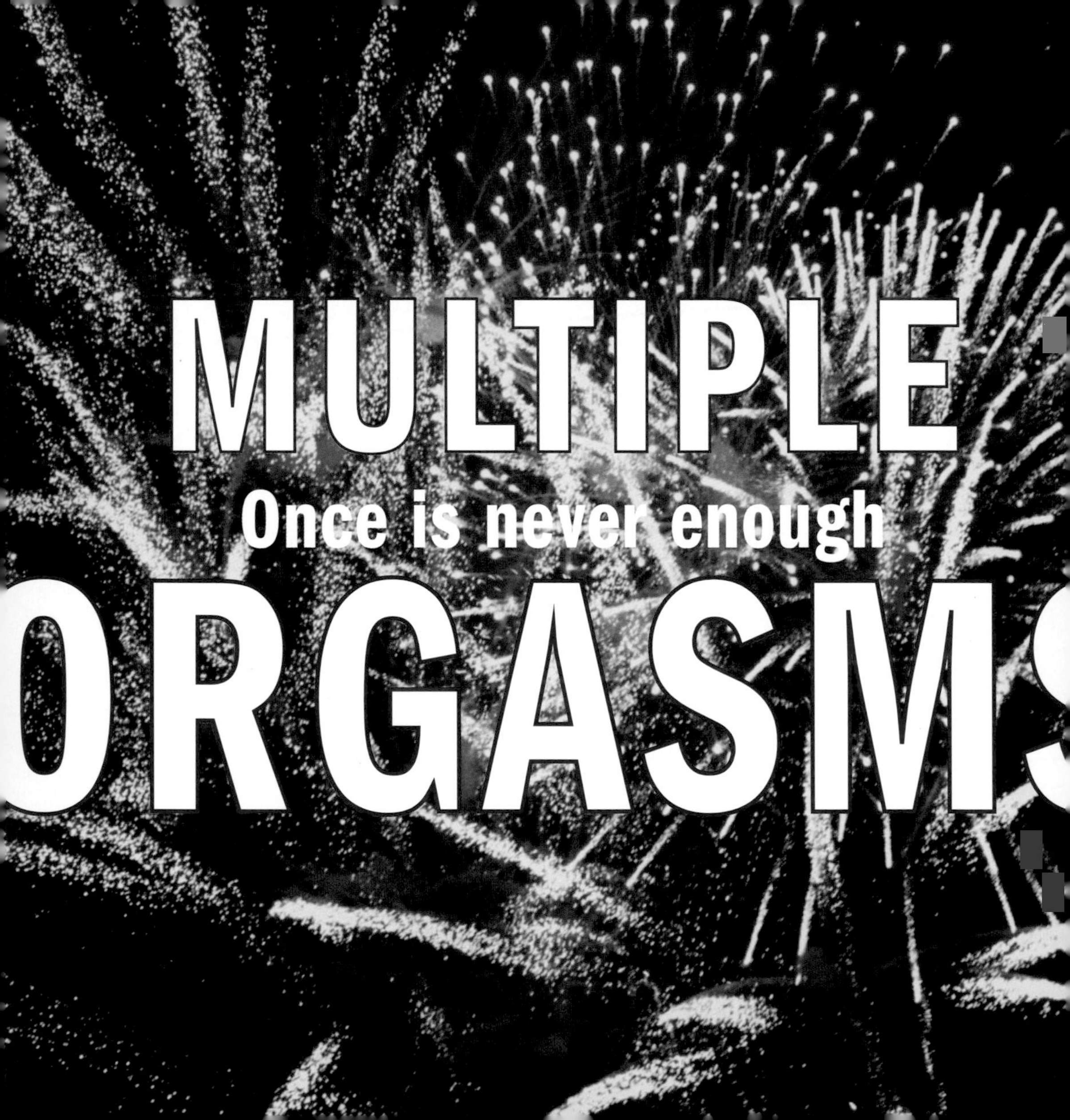

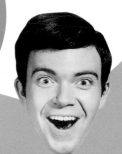

Unlearn
all of your bad tricks.
It's not necessary to ejaculate to experience a satisfying orgasm. Practice bringing yourself just to the edge of "popping." Immediately stop and let your arousal diminish. Then try it all over again. What's the rush?

Go
for the squeeze.
Play with yourself (or invite your favorite partner to assist) until you feel you're about to come. Squeeze the tip of your penis tightly with two or three fingers until the urge subsides. Start stroking again. Squeeze. You get the idea.

Women aren't the only ones having all the fun. While most men think of orgasms as a one-shot deal, plenty of hip (and very happy) guys are experiencing six and more orgasms during one love-making session. Here's how.

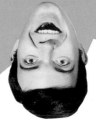

Do
your Kegel exercises.
Start strengthening your pubococcygeus (PC) muscles by stopping your urine in midstream about five times whenever you pee. By contracting the PC just before climax, men can experience multiple mini-orgasms followed by a Richter-worthy ejaculation.

Tug
your testicles.
By pulling your testicles down or holding them between your legs, ejaculations can be effectively delayed. (Best not to have the cameras rolling during your first few practice sessions.)

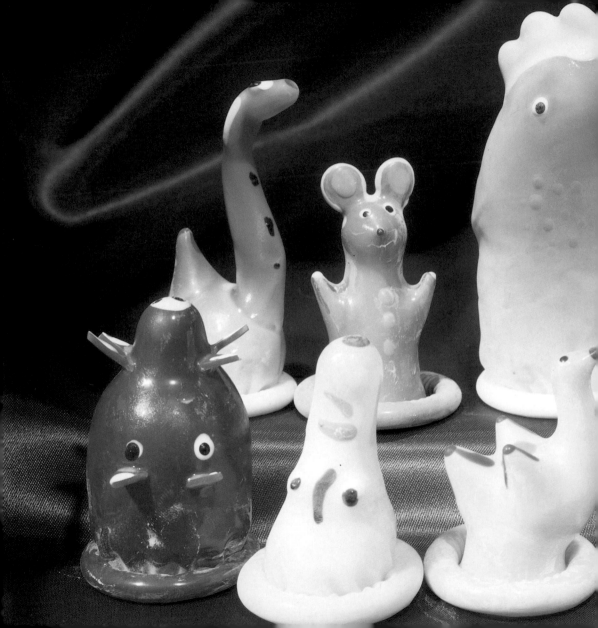

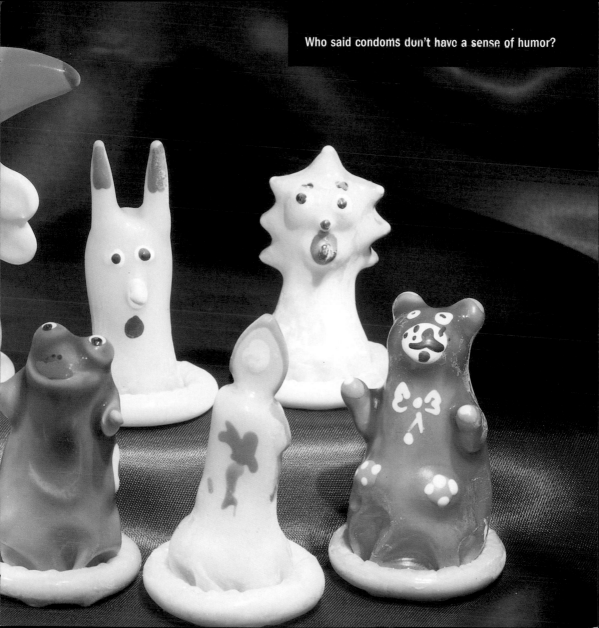

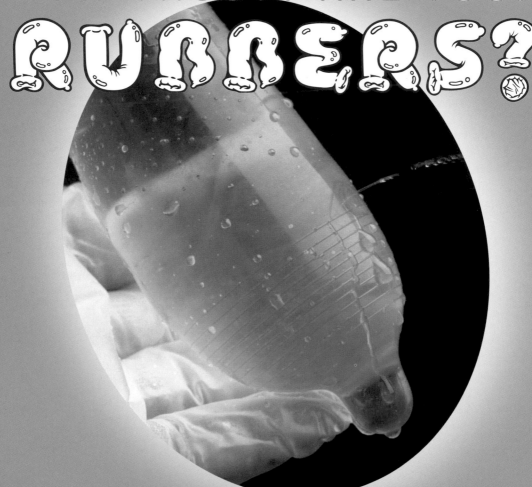

The news is shocking!

Among prophylactic testers, there's only one mantra: It's got to be perfect or out it goes. (Perhaps the condom industry could have a nice little chat with the automobile industry.) The biggest players in the global condom empire are sticklers for perfection, adhering to the incredibly stringent quality guidelines of the International Standards Organization.

Test #1, The Shocker. Every condom coming off the assembly line is stretched over a metal form, then treated to a high voltage zap. In a split second, any micro weakness in the latex film is discovered and that condom is instantly rejected.

Test #2, The Big Bubble. Part science, part Bazooka. In this test of tensile strength and elasticity, samples from every new batch of condoms are filled with a fixed amount of air until they reach the bursting point. Samples that "pop" too quickly often lead to an entire production run being discarded.

Test #3, The Wet Dream. Condom samples are filled with 300 milliliters of water to test for leakage and suspended for three minutes. Next, they're rolled on blotting paper in search of moisture. Should a few dewy drops appear, chances are excellent that the complete batch will be scrapped.

Test #4, The Old Geezer. In this procedure, samples are artificially aged at high temperatures, so that their efficacy can be tested at the end of their "five year" shelf life. And the codgers that don't make the grade? No retirement home for them, just a visit to the dump.

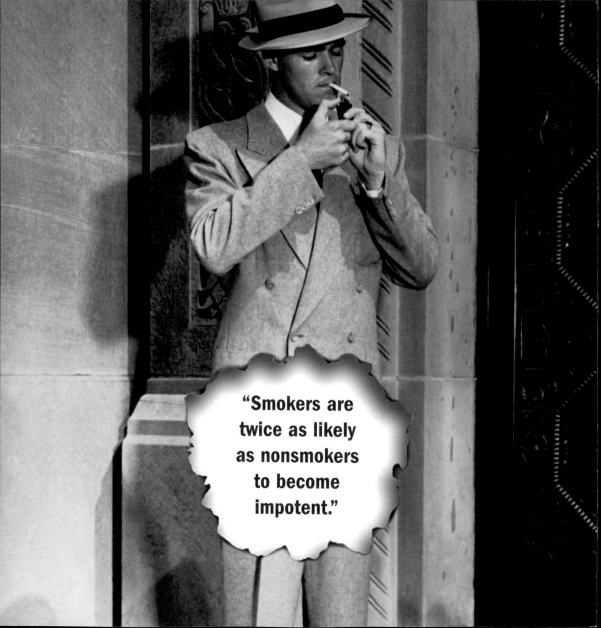

Erections—they're going up in smoke.

We've all seen the classic cliché from Hollywood: a couple lighting up after a fabulous round of lovemaking. Rather ironic, when you realize that smoking is one of the leading causes of impotence. And a prime player in reducing a man's fertility.

Medical studies confirm that smokers are twice as likely as nonsmokers to become impotent…a sobering fact that has yet to join the dire cigarette pack warnings most puffers prefer to ignore. Smoking damages the blood vessels in the penis, inhibiting the healthy flow of blood that leads to an erection. Since these vessels are considerably narrower than those leading to the heart, the penis is even more susceptible to the serious effects of smoking. A limp member is also recognized as an early warning sign that heart disease isn't too many ashtrays away.

Wait. There's a bright note in all this. While most smokers, especially those under age 30, refuse to quit over the potential damage to their hearts and lungs, the fear of giving up a satisfying sex life has seduced a substantial new wave of anti-nicotine converts. You decide: a pack or two a day. Or a lusty roll in the hay.

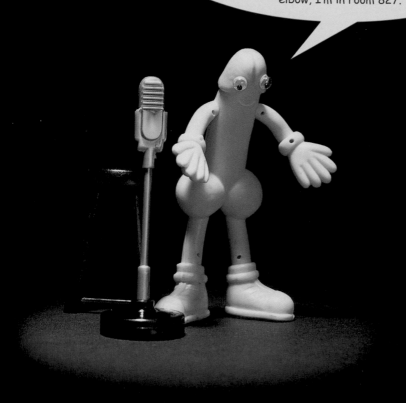

"At my age, I'm envious of a stiff wind."

RODNEY DANGERFIELD

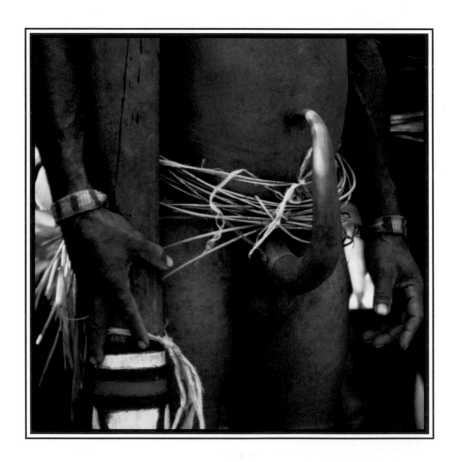

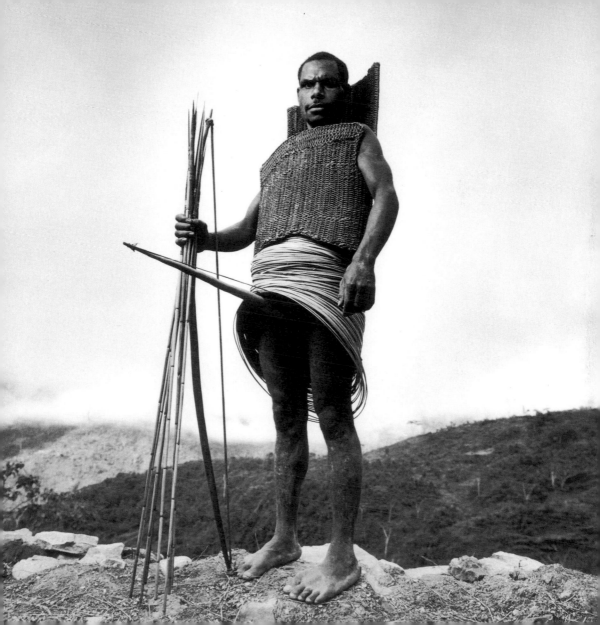

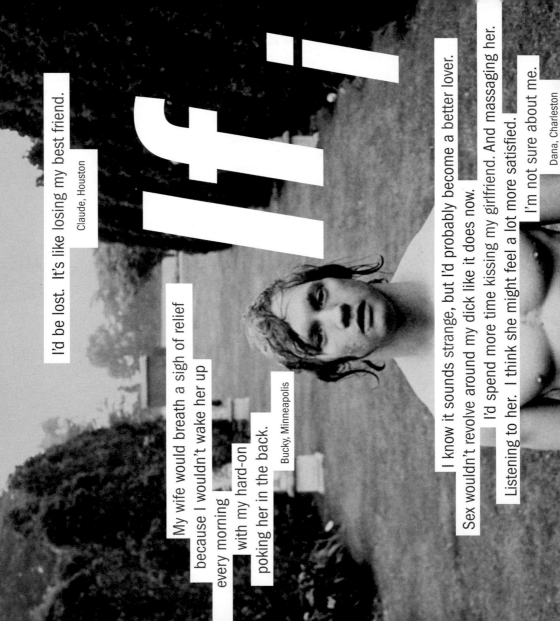

If

I'd be lost. It's like losing my best friend.

Claude, Houston

My wife would breath a sigh of relief because I wouldn't wake her up every morning with my hard-on poking her in the back.

Bucky, Minneapolis

I know it sounds strange, but I'd probably become a better lover. Sex wouldn't revolve around my dick like it does now. I'd spend more time kissing my girlfriend. And massaging her. Listening to her. I think she might feel a lot more satisfied. I'm not sure about me.

Dana, Charleston

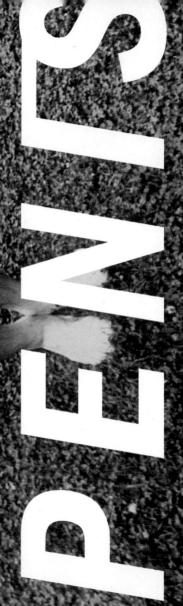

didn't HAVE a PENIS

What would I scratch?

Billy, Kenosha

I don't think I'd be as successful as I am today. Look, here's the way I see it: peckers and balls and testosterone and money are all linked together. No dick, no corner office. Does that make any sense?

Tom, Miami

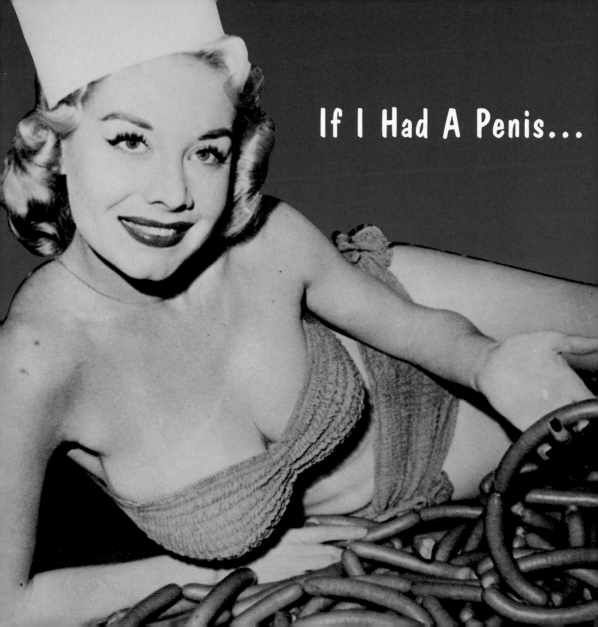

If I Had A Penis...

After a long meeting with a bunch of guys, I'd follow them into the men's room, stand at the urinal, whip it out and pee like the rest of them. Would they be shocked? Perhaps I'd only be confirming what some of them secretly suspected.

JEANETTE, CHICAGO

Very, very tenderly, I'd fuck my boyfriend up the ass.

TOBY, NEW YORK

The first thing I would do is make love to another woman. Jesus, it would almost be like fucking myself...knowing what really turns me on, sensing when it's time to go slow, faster, slower. Teasing with my cock. Wow!

HARRIET, LOS ANGELES

I'd get most excited about my balls. Big hairy balls, or I'd be disappointed. I'd shake them back and forth. Squeeze them into my laciest panties and let them hang out the sides. I'd have my cat lick them. Best of all, I'd watch my Romanian lady freak out as I spread my legs for my semi-annual bikini wax.

LYN, BOSTON

I'd pee in the woods. A lot. I've always wanted to do that.

REBECCA, SALT LAKE CITY

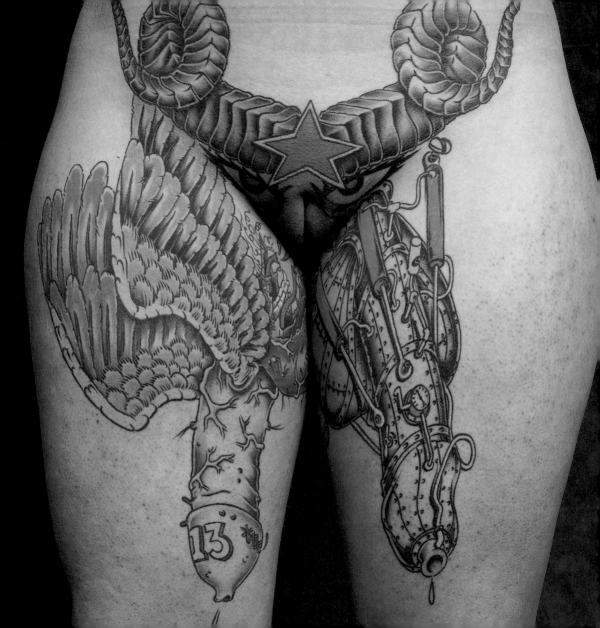

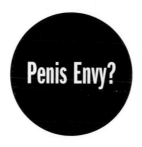

Penis Envy?

Sigmund Freud would be in his glory if this lady knocked on his Vienna door. By the early 1900s, the founder of psychoanalysis was convinced that little girls would reject their own genitals the moment they saw their father's or brother's penis. Girls, Freud expounded, were extremely envious of the male member, believing that their own penises had been castrated by their mothers. Searching for her long-lost penis, a girl would ultimately attach herself to her father. Later, she might find some comfort in the intact penises of other men in her life.

Naturally, the all-male medical community of the time bought this Freudian folly hook, line and sinker. These days, if there's any penis envy still flourishing, it surely exists among men. Straight and gay. Guys are always checking out other guys in the locker room. "Jesus, look at the donkey dong on that little wimp!" And look at those hunks on the screen...in and out, in and out like the hydraulic pumps on the Queen Mary. "Dear God, just another inch or two. Please."

Do women prefer BIG DICKS?

Sure, plenty get totally turned on by size…a real-life "fill 'er up" fantasy. But the majority of women prefer the comfort of an average sized penis *and* a sensitive lover who knows what to do with it. Since most of a woman's sexual pleasure comes from her clitoris and the outer two inches of her vagina (which contain most of the nerve endings), it's a thicker penis that ultimately has a lot more going for it.

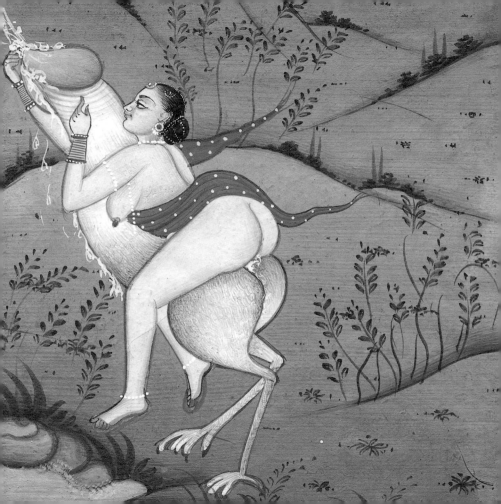

"Big Boy, Big Boy, oh give me all you've got," begged the empty milk bottle that I kept hidden in our storage bin in the basement, to drive wild after school with my vaselined upright. "Come, Big Boy, come," screamed the maddened piece of liver that in my own insanity, I bought one afternoon at a butcher shop and, believe it or not, violated behind a billboard on the way to a bar mitzvah lesson.

Philip Roth, *Portnoy's Complaint*

Aunt Miriam's "Absolutely Scrumptious" Chopped Liver

1 large onion - chopped

2 tablespoons yummy chicken fat (shmaltz)

1 pound chicken livers

salt and pepper

2 hard-boiled eggs finely chopped

additional chicken fat for flavoring

Heat half the shmaltz in a heavy skillet. Add liver and sauté until thoroughly cooked. Remove liver. Heat remaining shmaltz in same skillet over low heat. Add onions and cook until nice and soft.

Using a meat grinder, grind meat and onions. If you don't have a meat grinder you can use one of those fancy food processors. Remember, sweetheart, mixture should be coarse not creamy.

Transfer to a bowl. Stir in eggs. Give a taste. Add salt and pepper. (Your Uncle Izzy, may he rest in peace, always liked it when I added a little extra shmaltz.)

Servings: enough hors d'oeuvre schmears for 12

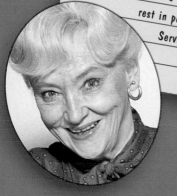

More Oysters, Casanova?

"I have loved women to a frenzy" wrote Giacomo Casanova (1725-1798) in his 12-volume memoirs, *History of My Life*. He was a soldier, magician, gambler, spy, a translator of the *Iliad*. But it is Casanova the tireless seducer who reigns supreme, crisscrossing the capitals of Europe in seach of fortune and lust…and the plumpest, freshest oysters that money could buy.

Oysters are the sea's legendary aphrodisiac. Casanova is reported to have consumed 50 of them every morning in the bath, accompanied by the damsel he fancied at the moment. Was it an oyster's vulva-on-the-half-shell imagery that stirred his loins? Or did he know that oysters are abundantly rich in zinc, a key ingredient in the production of sperm and testosterone?

"…we amused ourselves eating oysters, exchanging them when we already had them in our mouths. She gave me hers on her tongue, while I brought mine to her lips; there is no more luscious or voluptuous game between two lovers…"

Giacomo Casanova, *History of My Life*

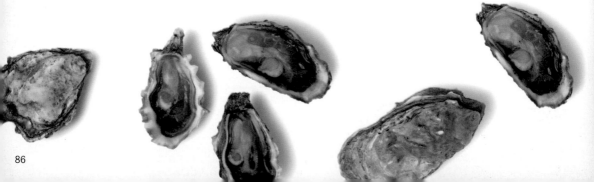

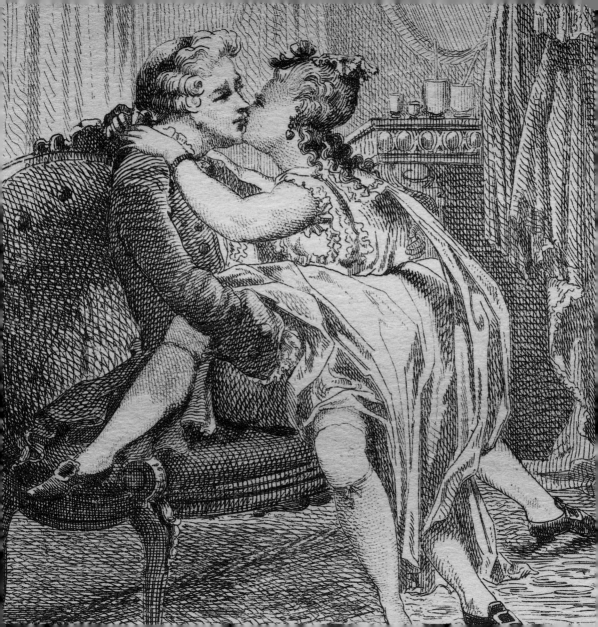

A FABULOUS HOME-COOKED MEAL
(WITH YOU FOR DESSERT)

YOUR LOVER SHAMPOOING YOUR HAIR

A QUICKIE IN AN ELEVATOR

24

A SLAP ACROSS THE ASS

GUARANTEED TURN-ONS

DIRTY TALK DURING SEX

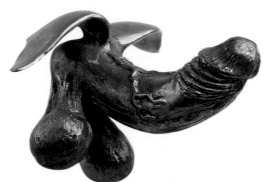

GETTING YOUR ARMPITS LICKED

A PERFECT SMILE

THE DELICIOUS MIX OF PERFUME AND SWEAT

HAVING YOUR UNDERWEAR RIPPED OFF

THREE-WAY SEX FOR THE FIRST TIME

A 90-MINUTE OUTDOOR MASSAGE

THE THRILL OF AN AFFAIR

MAKING LOVE IN A HAMMOCK

LETTING THE NEIGHBORS WATCH YOU
IN ACTION

THE LUXURIOUS EMBRACE OF LINEN SHEETS

A LUSTY PROPOSAL WHISPERED IN YOUR EAR

MAKING LOVE BY A BLAZING FIRE

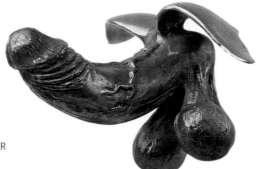

MOANS AND MORE MOANS

A WANDERING TOE

UNDRESSING YOUR LOVER
VERY, VERY SLOWLY

THE SOUND OF A WAILING SAXOPHONE

MAKING LOVE IN THE DUNES

A KISS THAT NEVER ENDS

A BAG-FUL OF NAUGHTY TOYS

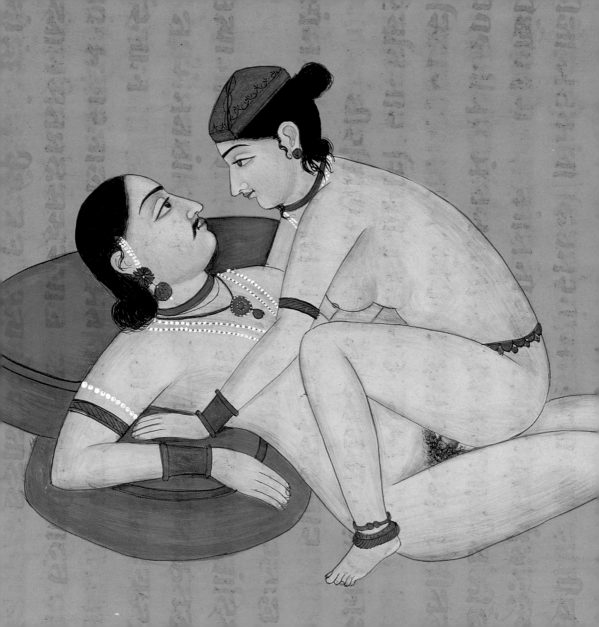

"*Then Bahloul inserted his member into the vagina of the Sultan's daughter, and she, settling down upon his engine, allowed it to penetrate entirely into her furnace till nothing more could be seen of it, not the slightest trace...She then gave herself up to an up-and-down dance, moving her bottom like a riddle; to the right and left, and forward and backward; never was there such a dance as this.*"

Sir Richard F. Buron's translation of *Perfumed Garden of Sheik Nefzaoui*

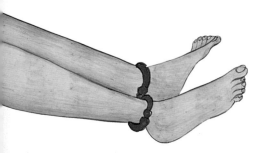

THOSE WILD AND CRAZY GREEKS

Think Wedgwood and Tupperware with a XXX rating, and you'll understand why some of the friskiest vases and urns from ancient Greece are just emerging from the back rooms of the world's great museums.

The phallus was the very symbol of life and the heart of Greece's decorative arts. The ideal penis was uncircumcised. And surprisingly small...a sure indicator of fertility, according to Aristotle, because the seminal seed had less distance to travel on its way to the uterus.

As you might imagine, the Greeks had grand phallic panoramas for every sexual appetite. Vases are adorned with supple young athletes, their foreskins pulled over the glans and tied with a leather string. (A practice called infibulation, in case you're interested.) Satyrs with huge erections can be observed chasing after prostitutes. Lonely wives are test-driving the newest dildos from Miletus, the dildo capital of the Hellenic age. Group orgies twist around spouts and handles. And platters sizzle with married men caressing their young male lovers.

The facts of life. For the ancient Greeks, they were as close as the china cabinet.

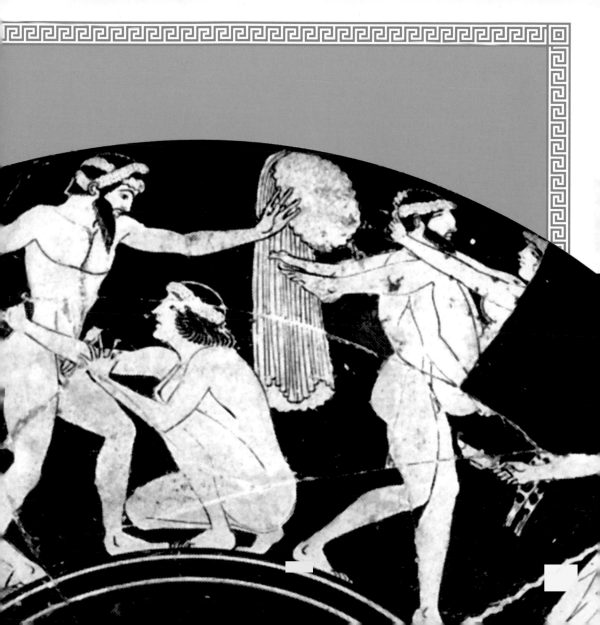

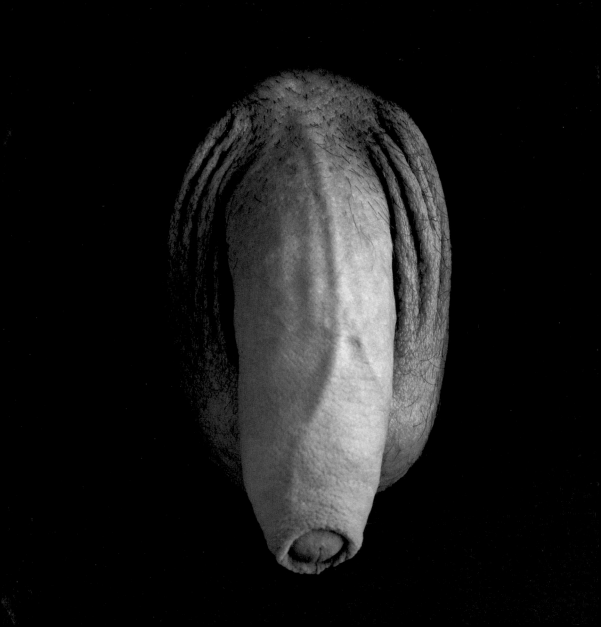

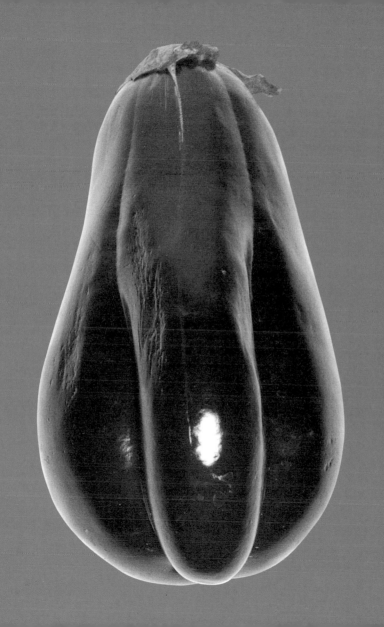

There's a lot more to Japan
than karaoki bars, Louis Vuitton boutiques
and bustling Toyota assembly lines. There's
also a world of eye-opening tradition.

HOUNEN MATSURI

E ach year on March 15, residents of tiny Komaki, about
250 miles south of Tokyo, celebrate a unique fertility festival called
Hounen Matsuri. The mile-long processional route to the shinto shrine of Tagata
Jinja echoes with the sounds of bamboo flutes, saki-satisfied onlookers and the
"hoh-sho hoh-sho" chant of men carrying a giant erect penis. The mighty specimen
shown here was carved from a single cypress tree trunk
by a 90-year-old man. A woody, in every sense of the
word, this 900 pound mega-phallus will be offered at
the shrine as a symbolic prayer for *hounen*, a fruitful year
of abundant harvests and growth for all living things.

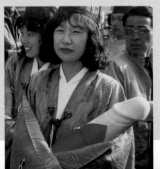

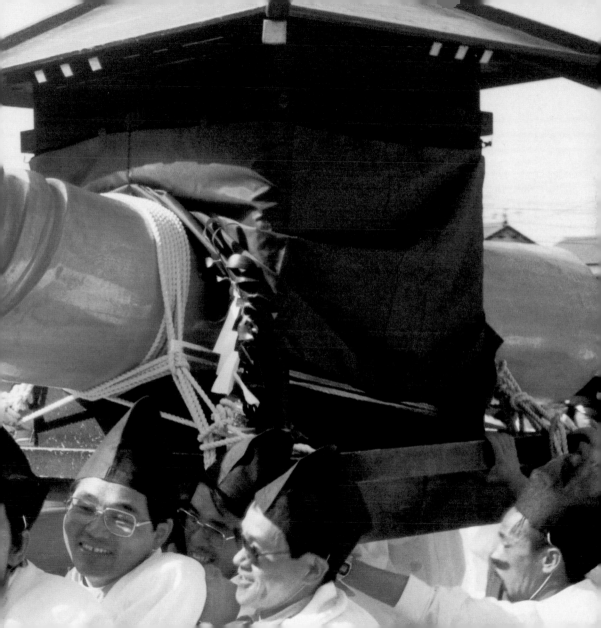

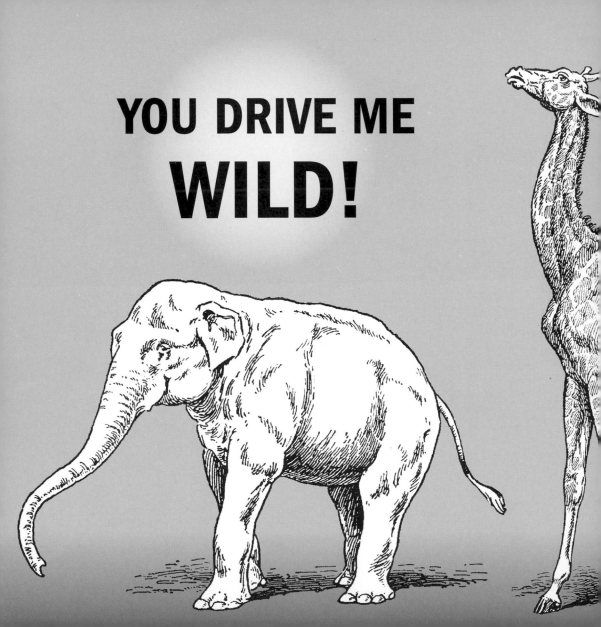

Gorillas may top the scales at 600 pounds, but their erect penises bottom out at around two inches. They don't get to use them much, maybe once a year, since females are in heat only a few days every four years.

Whales sport mega penises of nine feet, making them the real sharks of the deep. They mate once a year, keeping their hoses tucked inside their abdomens between performances.

Pigs' genitals are nature's corkscrews, with a twist that spirals up to 18 inches. This is what we call screwing...no sow ever has to ask, "Are you in yet?"

If your erection was four feet long and 100 pounds, you'd drag it on the ground, too. An **elephant's** penis has a built-in thrusting mechanism, so its owner can gracefully balance his forelegs on his ladyfriend's backside while his pecker does the work. Sex takes less than a minute. Gestation lasts 22 months.

Rising 19 feet and sporting a 24-inch erection, the male **giraffe** knows how to stand out in a crowd. After he shoots his load, he's off with his buddies, having nothing to do with his paramour du jour or her future offspring.

Talk about independence. An **octopus's** penis resides on one of his eight tentacles. When it's time to mate, the entire penis arm detaches and tracks down a female. After copulation, the penis dies, but remains attached to the female.

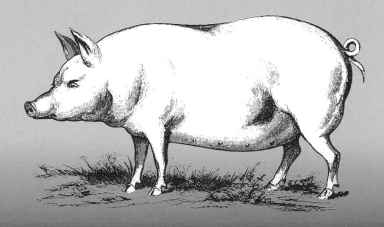

AN INTERVIEW WITH

CYNTHIA PLASTER CASTER

SHE TURNED ROCK 'N' ROLL
INTO HARD ROCK

She was a rock 'n' roll legend of the late sixties. And she's got the golden—make that plaster—oldies to prove it. Cynthia Plaster Caster made the pages of *Rolling Stone* because she had the ballsy audacity to ask superstars like Jimi Hendrix, The Lovin' Spoonful, Savoy Brown and Led Zeppelin if she could make a plaster cast of their erect penises. (It didn't matter that she had no idea what she was doing at first). Eventually, Cythia got the hang of well-hung rocksters. Today, she's back casting her favorite subject. Even has a little stand-up act recounting her wild adventures.

PENIS BOOK: What inspired you to cast famous dicks?

CYNTHIA PLASTER CASTER: My art professor in Chicago told us to cast something that was hard. All these rock stars from England were visiting here wearing real tight trousers with these big bulges. I just had to see what was inside.

PENIS BOOK: Had you ever seen a penis before?

CYNTHIA PLASTER CASTER: No. The first one I saw looked like a long snake...scared me shitless!

PENIS BOOK: How did Hendrix react when his pubic hair got stuck in your mold material?

CYNTHIA PLASTER CASTER: He was very patient. I forgot to lubricate his balls enough, so I had to pull his pubic hairs out one by one. He didn't complain at all.

PENIS BOOK: Tell us about the "plater."

CYNTHIA PLASTER CASTER: That's Cockney slang for a blow job. My girlfriend would come along with me to the person's hotel room and suck a guy to get him hard while I was mixing up all the casting stuff.

PENIS BOOK: The group Kiss even wrote a song about you...

CYNTHIA PLASTER CASTER: Yeah, the words are like Plaster Caster, grab a hold of me faster...if you want to see my love, just ask her...I like the song now, but not when they wrote it. They wanted people to think they'd been done by me.

PENIS BOOK: This performance show you're doing...

CYNTHIA PLASTER CASTER: I call it Talkin' Dick. I bring along a couple of my favorite penis castings. I read passages from my journals. Answer questions. I'm getting phone calls from all over. People love to hear tales about famous dick.

PENIS BOOK: Where do you keep your penis collection?

CYNTHIA PLASTER CASTER: In my bank vault. I can tell which casting belongs to which perfomer just by looking at it. It's a little more difficult in the dark.

PENIS BOOK: Do you have a name for your penis family?

CYNTHIA PLASTER CASTER: Of course. I call them my sweet babies.

"The good thing about masturbation is that you don't have to dress up for it."

TRUMAN CAPOTE

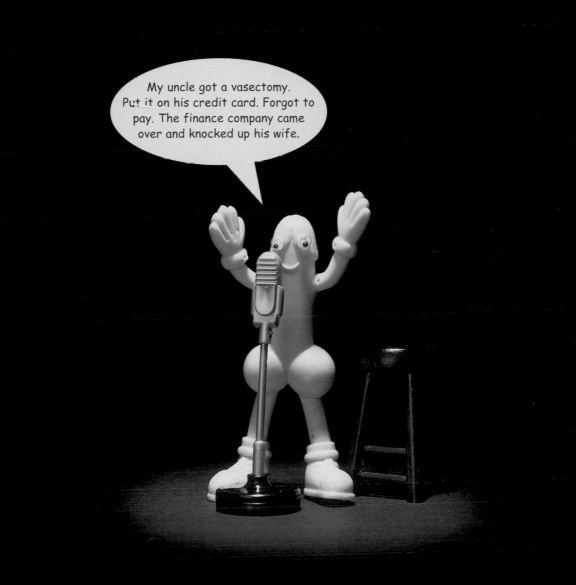

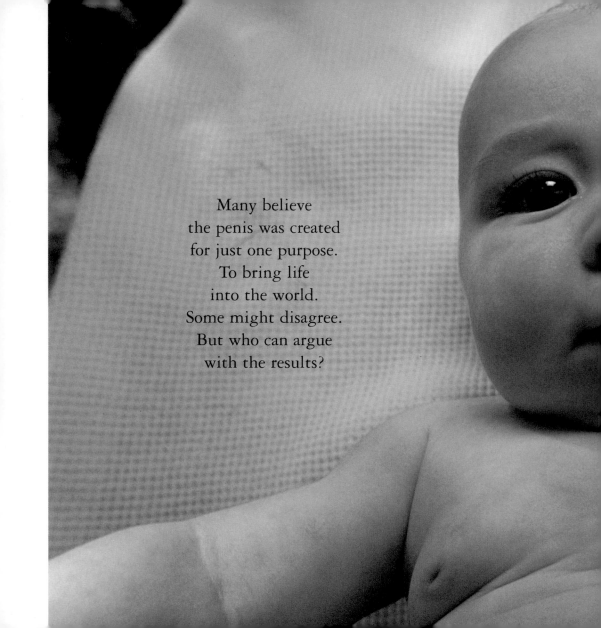

Many believe
the penis was created
for just one purpose.
To bring life
into the world.
Some might disagree.
But who can argue
with the results?

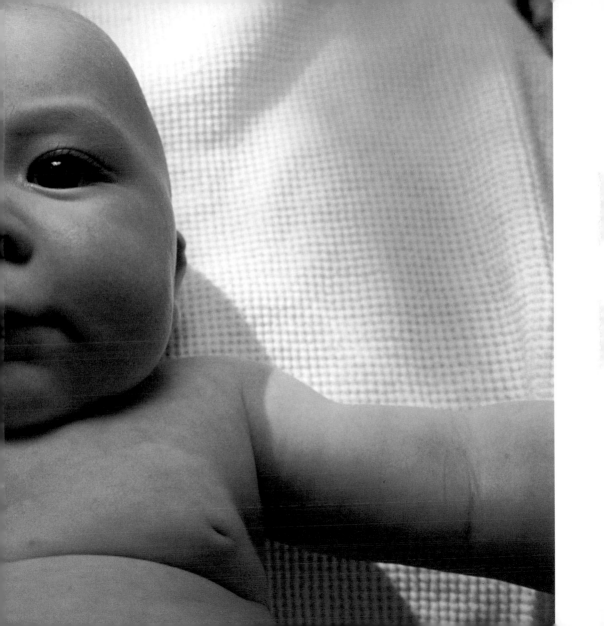

CREDITS

Cover, pp. 4-5, 26, 28-29, 32-34, 44, 52-53 & centerfold, 55, 62-63, 72, 88-89, 103, back cover: Studio NYC

Opposite page 1: Lucien Barnes

p. 2: Reed Massengill *Dana Laughing*

pp. 4-5: Penis merchandise courtesy Jimsons Novelties, NYC

pp. 10, 16-17, 58: Harvey Redding

pp. 13, 15, 27, 32 (frame), 39-40, 43, 64, 70, 86, 104-105: PhotoDisc

pp. 19-20 (left to right): Erich Lessing/Art Resource, NY (stone relief phallus, Pompeii), SuperStock (standing figure, Zaire), private collection (Peruvian fertility god), Erich Lessing/Art Resource, NY (Egyptian pre-dynastic figure), CORBIS/Penny Tweedie (Australian aboriginal rock painting)

p. 20: Sandi Fellman *Taboo*, from her book *The Japanese Tattoo* from Abbeville Press, a source of information for this spread

Following artwork courtesy Edie Solow of Erotics Gallery, NYC: p. 26 (painted Vienna bronze frogs c. 1890), p.55 (contemporary Hong Kong ivory netsuke), p.87 (engraving for Casanove in Bildern by Barraud c. 1936), pp. 88-89 (Winged Phallus by Doug Johns c. 1980), p. 90 (mid 20th century Indian painting)

pp. 30-31: ©1989 Estate of Tseng Kwong Chi and the Estate of Keith Haring

pp. 32-33: Hopping penises courtesy The Pleasure Chest, www.apleasurechest.com

p. 37: *Aperture f8* © Carlos Quiroz, courtesy Leslie-Lohman Gay Art Foundation, NYC, www.planet.net/corp/leslie_lohman — major thanks to Sal and Wayne, your doors were always open

p. 94: *Orchis* © Carlos Quiroz, courtesy Degen-Scharfman, NYC

p. 46: Early 1900s advertising courtesy of Bob McCoy, the Museum of Questionable Medical Devices, www.mtn.org/quack.com

p. 47: SuperStock

p. 49: Irwin Olaf *Joy* courtesy Wessell O'Connor Gallery, NYC — thanks to John and Billy, www.wesselloconnor.com

p. 60: Andreas Sterzing

pp. 62-63: Billy © Totem International, www.billyworld.com

p. 65, 85: Ewing Galloway

pp. 66-67: Nicholas Eveleigh

p. 68: Picture Quest

p. 74: CORBIS/ Charles & Josette Lenars (man in Papua, New Guinea)

p. 75: CORBIS/Chris Rainier (man in Highlands of Irian Jaya, Indonesia)

pp. 76-77: Arthur Tress *Hermaphrodite*

pp. 78: FPG International

p. 80: © 1998 William DeMichele

p. 83: Private collection (contemporary Indian painting in the Moghul manner)

p. 84: From *Portnoy's Complaint* by Philip Roth, Copyright © 1969 by Philip Roth. Reprinted by permission of Random House, Inc. For British Commonwealth distrubution: Copyright © 1969 by Philip Roth. Reprinted with the permission of The Wylie Agency, Inc., Inc

p. 95: Frank Degen *Eggplant I*, courtesy Degen-Scharfman, NYC

pp. 96-97: Peter Thoeny, with thanks for the information provided by his web site

pp. 100-101: Katrina Wittkamp

THANK YOU SO MUCH

Elaine. For your calls, encouragement and
your smiling Kentucky charm.

Tom, Chris and Cristina at Tom Dolle Design,
NYC. You brought these pages to life.
www.dolledesign.com

Edie Solow of Erotics Gallery, NYC.
Art has never been so tempting, or so
generously shared.
www.eroticsgallery.com

Mom. I'll always remember your asking:
"Why would anyone do a book
about peanuts?"

Jeanette. My fabulous friend and
Windy City proofreader.

Toby. Of course. For always being there.

THE PENIS BOOK WANTS YOU

Visit us at www.thepenisbook.com
It's the ultimate penis-info site.
Filled with ever-changing surprises.

E-mail us at veryfresh@aol.com
We wrote the book. But we don't
know it all. Talk to us.

Old fashioned? Write us at
Fresh Ideas Daily
Post Office Box 1
New York, NY 10276-0001